Sleep: A Very Short Introduction

Very Short Introductions available now:

ACCOUNTING Christopher Nobes
ADVERTISING Winston Fletcher
AFRICAN AMERICAN RELIGION
    Eddie S. Glaude Jr
AFRICAN HISTORY
    John Parker and Richard Rathbone
AFRICAN RELIGIONS Jacob K. Olupona
AGNOSTICISM Robin Le Poidevin
AGRICULTURE Paul Brassley and
    Richard Soffe
ALEXANDER THE GREAT Hugh Bowden
ALGEBRA Peter M. Higgins
AMERICAN HISTORY Paul S. Boyer
AMERICAN IMMIGRATION
    David A. Gerber
AMERICAN LEGAL HISTORY
    G. Edward White
AMERICAN POLITICAL HISTORY
    Donald Critchlow
AMERICAN POLITICAL PARTIES AND
    ELECTIONS L. Sandy Maisel
AMERICAN POLITICS Richard M. Valelly
THE AMERICAN PRESIDENCY
    Charles O. Jones
THE AMERICAN REVOLUTION
    Robert J. Allison
AMERICAN SLAVERY
    Heather Andrea Williams
THE AMERICAN WEST Stephen Aron
AMERICAN WOMEN'S HISTORY
    Susan Ware
ANAESTHESIA Aidan O'Donnell
ANARCHISM Colin Ward
ANCIENT ASSYRIA Karen Radner
ANCIENT EGYPT Ian Shaw
ANCIENT EGYPTIAN ART AND
    ARCHITECTURE Christina Riggs
ANCIENT GREECE Paul Cartledge
THE ANCIENT NEAR EAST
    Amanda H. Podany
ANCIENT PHILOSOPHY Julia Annas
ANCIENT WARFARE Harry Sidebottom
ANGELS David Albert Jones
ANGLICANISM Mark Chapman
THE ANGLO-SAXON AGE John Blair
THE ANIMAL KINGDOM Peter Holland
ANIMAL RIGHTS David DeGrazia
THE ANTARCTIC Klaus Dodds
ANTISEMITISM Steven Beller
ANXIETY Daniel Freeman and
    Jason Freeman
THE APOCRYPHAL GOSPELS Paul Foster
ARCHAEOLOGY Paul Bahn
ARCHITECTURE Andrew Ballantyne
ARISTOCRACY William Doyle
ARISTOTLE Jonathan Barnes

ART HISTORY Dana Arnold
ART THEORY Cynthia Freeland
ASTROBIOLOGY David C. Catling
ASTROPHYSICS James Binney
ATHEISM Julian Baggini
AUGUSTINE Henry Chadwick
AUSTRALIA Kenneth Morgan
AUTISM Uta Frith
THE AVANT GARDE David Cottington
THE AZTECS David Carrasco
BACTERIA Sebastian G. B. Amyes
BARTHES Jonathan Culler
THE BEATS David Sterritt
BEAUTY Roger Scruton
BESTSELLERS John Sutherland
THE BIBLE John Riches
BIBLICAL ARCHAEOLOGY Eric H. Cline
BIOGRAPHY Hermione Lee
BLACK HOLES Katherine Blundell
THE BLUES Elijah Wald
THE BODY Chris Shilling
THE BOOK OF MORMON Terryl Givens
BORDERS Alexander C. Diener and
    Joshua Hagen
THE BRAIN Michael O'Shea
BRICS Andrew F. Cooper
THE BRITISH CONSTITUTION
    Martin Loughlin
THE BRITISH EMPIRE Ashley Jackson
BRITISH POLITICS Anthony Wright
BUDDHA Michael Carrithers
BUDDHISM Damien Keown
BUDDHIST ETHICS Damien Keown
BYZANTIUM Peter Sarris
CANCER Nicholas James
CAPITALISM James Fulcher
CATHOLICISM Gerald O'Collins
CAUSATION Stephen Mumford and
    Rani Lill Anjum
THE CELL Terence Allen and Graham Cowling
THE CELTS Barry Cunliffe
CHAOS Leonard Smith
CHEMISTRY Peter Atkins
CHILD PSYCHOLOGY Usha Goswami
CHILDREN'S LITERATURE
    Kimberley Reynolds
CHINESE LITERATURE Sabina Knight
CHOICE THEORY Michael Allingham
CHRISTIAN ART Beth Williamson
CHRISTIAN ETHICS D. Stephen Long
CHRISTIANITY Linda Woodhead
CITIZENSHIP Richard Bellamy
CIVIL ENGINEERING David Muir Wood
CLASSICAL LITERATURE William Allan
CLASSICAL MYTHOLOGY Helen Morales
CLASSICS Mary Beard and John Henderson

For more information visit our web site
www.oup.com/vsi/

Steven W. Lockley and Russell G. Foster

SLEEP
A Very Short Introduction

OXFORD
UNIVERSITY PRESS

OXFORD
UNIVERSITY PRESS

Great Clarendon Street, Oxford OX2 6DP

Oxford University Press is a department of the University of Oxford.
It furthers the University's objective of excellence in research, scholarship,
and education by publishing worldwide in

Oxford New York

Auckland Cape Town Dar es Salaam Hong Kong Karachi
Kuala Lumpur Madrid Melbourne Mexico City Nairobi
New Delhi Shanghai Taipei Toronto

With offices in

Argentina Austria Brazil Chile Czech Republic France Greece
Guatemala Hungary Italy Japan Poland Portugal Singapore
South Korea Switzerland Thailand Turkey Ukraine Vietnam

Oxford is a registered trade mark of Oxford University Press
in the UK and in certain other countries

Published in the United States
by Oxford University Press Inc., New York

British Library Cataloguing in Publication Data

Data available

Library of Congress Cataloging in Publication Data

Library of Congress Control Number: 2011945235

Typeset by SPI Publisher Services, Pondicherry, India
Printed in Great Britain
on acid-free paper by
Ashford Colour Press Ltd, Gosport, Hampshire

ISBN 978-0-19-958785-8

9 10 8

This book is dedicated to:

SWL – to my parents, Barbara and Chris;
RGF – to Elizabeth, Charlotte, William, and Victoria.

Contents

Acknowledgements

We would like to thank the following people for their helpful comments on the manuscript: Francesco Cappuccio, Emma Cussans, Lawrence Epstein, Erin Flynn-Evans, Patrick Fuller, Sanjeev Kothare, Leon Kreitzman, Andrew Philips, Kate Porcheret, Katharina Wulff. We also thank Jayne Butters and Peter Strasser for helpful information.

List of illustrations

Chapter 1
Sleep through the ages

For centuries, we have regarded sleep as a simple suspension of activity, a passive state of unconsciousness, and for centuries we have been wrong. This failure to understand the active nature of sleep is perhaps one of the reasons why our 24/7 society has developed such little regard for it. At best, many of us tolerate the fact that we need to sleep, and at worst we think of sleep as an illness that needs a cure. This attitude, held by so many in business, politics, industry, and even the health profession, is not only unsustainable but potentially dangerous.

Our everyday experience tells us that a night of sleep has considerable benefits, and this subjective feeling is supported by an increasing body of scientific evidence – some of which we review in this book. Aside from making us feel better, sleep helps our brains find creative solutions to everyday problems. History is replete with incidents when scientists and artists have awoken to make their most notable contributions after long periods of frustration. Friedrich Kekulé came up with the chemical ring structure of benzene – the famous image of a snake biting its tail; Otto Loewi developed his principle of chemical neurotransmission – for which he received a Nobel Prize; Dmitri Mendeleev ordered the chemical elements into the periodic table. In the arts, Robert Louis Stevenson had his inspiration for *The Strange Case of*

Dr Jekyell and Mr Hyde after sleeping; likewise, Samuel Taylor Coleridge's poem *Kubla Khan* was supposed to have come to him in a dream – albeit an opium-fuelled one – as was Giuseppe Tartini's violin sonata 'Devil's Trill'. Salvador Dali was obsessed with the creative potential of sleep; and Richard Wagner, perhaps more than any other artist, used sleep to both inspire his composition and provide a dominant theme in his operas.

Our treatment of sleep today is brutish. Adults, on average, sleep about 7 hours a night, with 5% sleeping fewer than 5 hours, and 6% sleeping more than 9 hours (Figure 1). By contrast, some historical reports suggest that we slept significantly longer in the past. During the long nights of winter, sleep probably occurred for extended periods of time with two or sometimes more discrete bouts of sleep separated by intervals of resting wakefulness. In pre-industrial times, we may have slept up to 10 hours a day, depending on the season. Modern-day experiments support these ideas: if people are kept on a winter schedule (long nights, short days), they do sleep more than when kept on a summer pattern. If subjects are given very long opportunities to sleep, they will eventually reach a stable sleep duration of about 8.5 hours in young adults, and 7.5 hours in older adults, more than most people currently get. The introduction of electric lighting in the 19th century, and the restructuring of work hours and social schedules caused by industrialization, have meant that our species has become progressively detached from the natural 24-hour cycles of light and dark (see Chapters 8 and 9).

It seems likely that we sleep less now than at any other time in our recent history. Most data collected from industrial nations over the past 50 years show a general decline in sleep in line with the culture of long work hours, more shift-work, long commutes, global communication across multiple time zones, and freedom from many economic and social constraints. These factors and the 24-hour availability of almost everything have conspired to

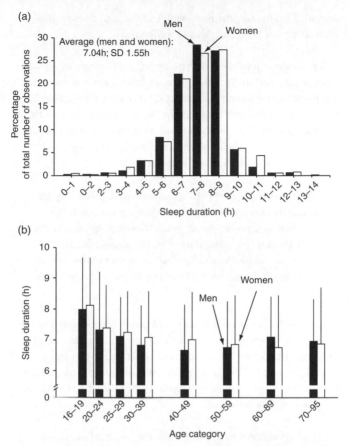

1. **Sleep in Britain, from a 2003 survey of about 2,000 British adults.**
(a) shows that average sleep duration is around 7 hours per night, with
5% sleeping fewer than 5 hours and 6% sleeping more than 9 hours;
(b) shows the changes in sleep duration with age and between men and
women

demote sleep in our priorities, which, as we shall discuss, has come at a price to our health and wellbeing.

Before we delve into the modern-day science of sleep, we should place our current understanding into a brief historical context. Sleep has been studied for at least 2,500 years, with the Greek philosophers/physicians Alcmaeon, Hippocrates, and Aristotle all putting forward theories on the causes and functions of sleep. In 350 BC, Aristotle wrote a volume entitled *On Sleep and Sleeplessness*, and the opening text reads:

> With regard to sleep and waking, we must consider what they are: whether they are peculiar to soul or to body, or common to both; and if common, to what part of soul or body they appertain: further, from what cause it arises that they are attributes of animals, and whether all animals share in them both, or some partake of the one only, others of the other only, or some partake of neither and some of both.

These questions, perhaps slightly rephrased, framed much of the debate about sleep for the next 2,000 years. Yet we have to wait until the 20th century for modern sleep science to emerge formally, prompted by Henri Pieron, who published the first text to consider the physiology of sleep in 1913, entitled *Le Probleme Physiologique du Sommeil*.

Early observations on sleep often put the source of sleepiness within the stomach, with the idea that warm vapours arose from the gut during digestion to initiate sleep, and that different foods could influence sleepiness. In the early 17th century, René Descartes suggested the brain as the organ mediating sleep and wake states, with the pineal gland (the site of melatonin production – see Chapter 2) controlling the flow of 'animal spirits' around the brain. Many theories regarding the origin of sleep were postulated in the 18th and 19th centuries, including the presence of a 'sleep substance' or toxin which built up during the day and dissipated at night; that sleepiness was affected by blood flow; or that nerve cells were paralysed at night and could not communicate – concepts that are still being explored today.

The idea that the brain was central to sleep was developed at the start of the 19th century with experiments on birds by Luigi Rolando and later by Jean Pierre Flourens, who showed that a permanent sleepiness was induced in the birds after removal of their cerebral hemispheres. It would be another century or so before the site of the sleep centres could be identified in humans. This advance was primarily due to the observations of Constantin von Economo, a Romanian psychiatrist, made during the catastrophic influenza epidemic of 1918. He noted that some of his patients with viral encephalitis showed either insomnia (lack of sleep) or excessive sleepiness (encephalitis lethargic). Based on the damage he found when examining the brains of dead patients, von Economo proposed that the brain contained different areas that regulate sleep and wakefulness. He suggested that because damage in the anterior hypothalamus caused prolonged insomnia, this region of the brain normally produced sleep. By contrast, he found that damage to the lateral/posterior hypothalamus caused prolonged sleepiness, and so concluded that this region was responsible for wakefulness. A little under a hundred years later, he was proved correct, as we shall discuss in Chapter 3.

A major technological advance in the science of sleep was the ability to measure brain activity during sleep. The first human electroencephalogram (EEG) was performed by Hans Berger in 1928 after improvements in electrophysiology allowed him to place electrodes on the human scalp to record the electrical activity of the brain (rather than on the brain directly), and to demonstrate differences between sleep and awake states (see Chapter 2). These methods still form the basis of most clinical sleep assessments today. These techniques prompted a rapid expansion in the study of sleep through the 20th century.

In 1939, the Russian sleep researcher Nathaniel Kleitman published *Sleep and Wakefulness*, a seminal text summarizing the knowledge of the day, which was revised in 1963. Kleitman established the first laboratory dedicated to sleep in 1925 at the University of Chicago and studied many aspects of sleep and sleep deprivation, including a famous experiment in which he and student Bruce Richardson lived for a month in Mammoth Caves in Kentucky and demonstrated daily rhythms in sleep and temperature in the absence of external influences. His most renowned contribution, however, was the formal description of rapid eye movement (REM) sleep after observations by his student, Eugene Aserinsky. While eye movements during sleep had been observed and reported for centuries, Aserinsky and Kleitman were the first to denote use of these eye movements in the formal characterization of different sleep subtypes.

Around the same time – the 1940s and 1950s – researchers, including Giuseppe Moruzzi, Horace Magoun, and Michel Jouvet, advanced the work of von Economo and showed that stimulation and lesions of different regions of another part of the brain – the brainstem – could greatly influence sleep. Furthermore, recordings from these regions changed markedly during sleep and wakefulness. Collectively, their work enabled these researchers to conclude that multiple structures within the brainstem are involved in maintaining wakefulness, and the generation of the NREM-REM cycle of sleep (Chapter 2).

These early pioneers established sleep as a serious subject worthy of study and created a new scientific field. Today, a search of 'PubMed', an electronic database of scientific articles maintained by the United States National Library of Medicine, recalls nearly 110,000 articles in a search for 'Sleep', and this number increases daily. Summarizing over 100,000 research articles in a small book is a challenge, but we hope that this *Very Short Introduction* will help guide readers into the fascinating world of sleep.

Chapter 2
Sleep generation and regulation – a framework

Even if we are not certain as to the exact function of sleep (Chapter 4), a great deal is understood about what happens to the brain and body during sleep. While sleep can be defined on the basis of behavioural changes, it is the ability to measure electrical activity patterns across the brain that has defined sleep in humans and other mammals.

The electroencephalogram (EEG)

The brain is assembled from billions of neurones that communicate with each other by electrical and chemical (neurotransmitter) signals. The collective interactions of these neurones give rise to voltage changes that can be recorded from the surface of the brain. Such recordings were first made in animals by Richard Canton towards the end of the 19th century and developed by Berger for human measurements – and the electroencephalogram, or EEG, was born. When two or more electrodes are placed on the scalp, the voltage between the electrodes can be recorded (Figure 2). Berger was able to show that when subjects were awake, the EEG showed a fast (high frequency) and small amplitude pattern of activity which became slower (lower frequency) and had larger amplitude waves as individuals drifted towards sleep (Figure 3). Building upon Berger's observations during the 1930s, discernible EEG sleep 'stages' were described by several researchers, and in 1953 Kleitman and Aserinsky described what is now known as rapid eye movement (REM) sleep. By the late 1960s, Allan Rechtschaffen and Anthony Kales had formalized the characterization of sleep stages on the basis of different EEG patterns.

There are two distinct types of sleep – rapid eye movement (REM) and non-rapid eye movement (NREM) sleep – which alternate to form a NREM–REM sleep cycle approximately every 90 to 100 minutes (Figure 4). Depending on the duration of sleep, there are on average four to five sleep cycles per night, and visualization of the entire sleep episode is termed the 'hypnogram'. As shown in Figure 3, NREM stage 1 is typified by theta waves, and this is also referred to as somnolence or drowsy sleep. Sudden twitches and jerks of the limbs may occur during this stage. NREM stage 2 is characterized by short bursts of activity called 'sleep spindles' and

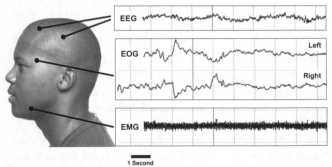

2. The electroencephalogram (EEG), electrooculogram (EOG), and electromyogram (EMG) can be recorded simultaneously from subjects by placing recording electrodes on the skin in the positions indicated. For EEG, multiple electrodes are usually employed – the number varies from eight to hundreds depending on the type of analysis required

high-amplitude and low-frequency events known as K-complexes. Muscular activity, as shown by an electromyogram, or EMG, decreases, whilst conscious awareness of the external environment disappears. NREM stages 3 and 4 are often called deep or slow-wave sleep (SWS) and are characterized by the presence of delta waves. This is the stage when parasomnias such as night terrors, bedwetting, sleep-walking, and sleep-talking occur. The amount of time spent in SWS is correlated with the amount of prior sleep deprivation (Chapter 4). During REM sleep, the beta EEG patterns are almost identical to those measured in a fully awake individual, which is why REM sleep is often called 'paradoxical sleep'.

The proportion of NREM and REM sleep in each cycle changes throughout the night, with higher levels of NREM stages 3 and 4 (slow-wave sleep, SWS) during the first few cycles and an increasing amount of REM sleep in later cycles (Figure 4). NREM sleep is generally associated with a more stable physiology – regular breathing patterns and lower heart rate – whereas REM sleep is a more active process with a more variable but generally higher breathing and heart rate, blood pressure, and blood flow to the brain. On average, about 25% of the human sleep episode will consist of REM sleep (Figure 3a). By definition, REM sleep is usually associated with rapid eye movements, detected by measuring the electrical activity generated by the muscles moving the eye using the electrooculogram (EOG). REM sleep is also accompanied by an inhibition of the skeletal muscles, termed 'atonia', and this is measured using electrodes placed near the chin. This is the electromyogram (EMG) (Figure 2).

Dreaming

Dreaming can occur in both NREM and REM sleep, but dreams in REM tend to be longer, more vivid, complex, and bizarre. Dreams are thought to span most of the REM episode and perhaps as much as 40% of NREM and occur in real time – the old idea that dreams occur in a flash when we wake is now not generally supported. A detailed discussion of dreams and dreaming is offered by J. Allan Hobson in *Dreaming: A Very Short Introduction*. Briefly, dream content is very variable but almost always involves the dreamer and usually individuals who are familiar to the dreamer. Dreams are almost always visual experiences and rarely involve taste or smell. If individuals have been blind since birth, dreams are dominated by sound, touch, and emotional feelings. Those who have lost their sight during childhood (around 7–8 years), however, have dreams dominated by visual experiences. Dreams are often deeply bizarre but usually draw from our experiences at some very basic level. A current theory is that dreaming is a by-product of the processing of information and the consolidation of memory.

Box 1: A curious feature of REM sleep

During REM sleep, males have nocturnal erections and females experience clitoral engorgement. These events have been studied most in males, in whom erections appear to last for most of the REM episode during night and day sleep. Erections have been recorded during REM in babies and even in individuals on life-support. There are even suggestions that the cave paintings in Lascaux in southern France depict sleeping males with pronounced erections. Sexual intercourse prior to sleep does not alter the level of penile tumescence in the subsequent sleep episode, and excessive alcohol consumption, which inhibits penile erection when awake, has little effect on its robustness. Other mammals such as rats and dogs have also been reported to show penile erections during REM. Although REM sleep is associated with our most vivid dreams, empirical studies suggest that no correlation exists between the sexual content of a dream and penile erection.

(a)

Sleep Stage Classification (Old)	Sleep Stage Classification (New)	% Time Asleep	Frequency HZ (cycles per second)	Amplitude μv (micro volts)	EEG Wave Type
Awake		N/A	>12	<30	beta
Relaxed		N/A	8–12	<50	alpha
Non-REM Stage 1	N1	5%	4–8	50–100	theta
Non-REM Stage 2	N2	45%	4–8	50–150	theta, spindles, K-complexes
Non-REM Stage 3	N3 Delta or Slow Wave Sleep (SWS)	12%	2–4	100–150	delta & theta
Non-REM Stage 4		13%	0.5–2	100–200	delta & theta
REM	REM	25%	>12	<30	beta

(b)

3. Adult human EEG patterns for different wake and sleep stages. (a) Column 1 of this table classifies sleep into non-rapid eye movement (NREM) and rapid eye movement (REM) sleep stages. In column 2, a recently introduced sleep classification scheme is listed which divides sleep into the broader categories of Wake, N1, N2, N3, and REM. The additional columns in (a) detail the EEG wave-forms and the time spent in different sleep states. (b) Illustrates the EEG traces that are used to define the different sleep states

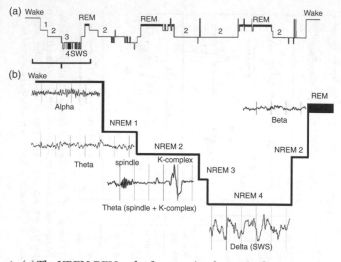

4. (a) The NREM-REM cycles for an entire sleep episode (hypnogram) are illustrated over 7 hours. The time spent in different EEG states varies considerably over the night. Slow-wave sleep (SWS) episodes tend to occur during the first half of the night, whilst REM sleep occurs more frequently during the second half of the night. Natural wake may occur after REM sleep, but not always. (b) A portion of the EEG profile (around 70 minutes) expanded from (a). The human EEG changes progressively from wake through sleep from low-amplitude and high-frequency patterns when awake to large-amplitude and low-frequency synchronous oscillations during slow-wave sleep (SWS) – NREM stage 3 and stage 4. From SWS, there is a rapid advance into NREM stage 2 and 1 before a period of REM sleep. The cycle then repeats approximately every 90 minutes

The two-process model of sleep–wake regulation

The two-process model of sleep regulation, first proposed by Alexander Borbély in 1982, provides a very useful way to think about sleep-wake timing. The model suggests that two oscillators contribute to sleep, an hourglass-like sleep–wake 'counter' and an internal 24-hour circadian rhythm of sleep and arousal. These two processes interact to determine the timing, duration, and structure of sleep (Figure 5). The hourglass counter describes the intuitive pattern of sleep – the likelihood of falling asleep depends on how long we have been awake; and the chances of waking up increase the longer we have been asleep. This seemingly simple concept is the homeostatic part of the two-process model, termed 'Process S', which 'counts' how long we have been asleep or awake and is a predictor of 'sleep pressure'; the longer you stay awake, the greater the build-up in sleep pressure (Figure 6). As we sleep, we reduce this sleep pressure until it becomes low enough to allow us to wake up. The amount of slow-wave sleep (SWS) in the sleep episode increases as the sleep pressure (Process S) increases, for example in response to sleep deprivation.

We also understand intuitively that it is generally easier to fall asleep at 12 midnight than it is to fall asleep at 12 midday. This is because there is a 24-hour rhythm in sleep propensity determined by an internal 24-hour clock in the brain, located in the suprachiasmatic nuclei (SCN) of the hypothalamus. Independently of any environmental signals, the circadian pacemaker (*circadian*, 'about a day') spontaneously generates near-24-hour rhythms which in turn control the timing of many rhythmic behavioural, physiological, and metabolic functions, including sleep propensity and sleep structure, temperature regulation, production of hormones such as melatonin and cortisol, cardiac and lung function, glucose and insulin levels, and many more. These endogenous near-24-hour rhythms are synchronized to the 24-hour day by daily environmental time cues, the most important of which is the 24-hour light–dark cycle. In the two-process model, the circadian pacemaker determines the 24-hour rhythm of sleep and arousal termed 'Process C' (Figure 6). The circadian clock and its regulation by light are considered in detail in Chapter 3.

Under normal circumstances, Processes S and C cycle in opposition to maintain wakefulness during the day and a long bout of consolidated sleep at night. The progressive increase in the

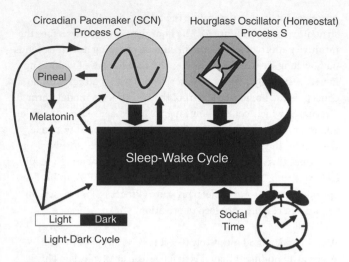

5. Diagram illustrating the key components and their interactions in the generation and maintenance of the sleep–wake cycle. Sleep is regulated by two broad mechanisms involving both the 24-hour body clock (circadian system; known as Process C) and a wake-dependent homeostatic build-up of sleep pressure (also called Process S). Sleep itself will feed back to regulate both Process C and Process S. Light plays a key role in synchronizing the circadian pacemaker, gated by the sleep–wake cycle, acutely suppressing melatonin production from the pineal, and in regulating levels of alertness. Social activities such as meal times or forced awakening by an alarm clock will also drive sleep–wake activity

circadian alerting signal through much of the day is counteracted by the increasing homeostatic pressure for sleep with increasing time awake. Conversely, the increasing circadian drive for sleep through the night is opposed by the reduction in homeostatic drive that occurs during sleep. Without the circadian drive for sleep, the sleep episode at night would be much shorter because sleep pressure dissipates rapidly during the first half of sleep. The underlying reason why some people are naturally long or short sleepers is not fully understood but is likely to be related to how the brain responds to the build-up of sleep pressure.

The worst of both worlds – awake for a long time at the wrong time

Under certain circumstances, Process S and Process C can interact to cause a dramatic increase in sleepiness that has enormous safety implications (see Chapters 8 and 9). If an individual has been awake for a long time (high sleep pressure) and also happens to be awake during the night, when the circadian system is strongly promoting sleep, a 'perfect storm' of sleepiness occurs. Under these conditions, the two processes interact in a way that makes sleepiness much worse than that predicted by simply adding their effects together. This non-linear interaction makes it particularly dangerous to be awake between 3 and 6 a.m., when the circadian rhythm of sleepiness is at its peak, coupled with a build-up of sleep pressure because of extended time awake (Figure 6). Such a situation is a common occurrence for shift-workers, doctors, firefighters, and other professionals who must be alert during normal sleeping hours, and this is a particularly vulnerable time for sleepiness-related accidents and injuries.

Sleep inertia – the problem of getting going in the morning

In addition to describing sleep timing and structure, the two-process model also describes the general time course of sleepiness and performance throughout the day. Sleepiness generally increases the longer you stay awake, but it is also mediated by a strong circadian rhythm which also affects general mood and the ability to concentrate, remember, and react. Under normal sleep–wake conditions, daytime performance is relatively stable before declining towards the end of the day, as predicted with longer time awake. The two-process model, however, would also predict the highest alertness at the end of sleep, when sleep pressure has been maximally reduced. Personal experience, however, tells us that this is not the case, and that there is a third process that explains our grogginess when we first wake up – sleep inertia, or 'Process W' (Figure 6). In fact, it can take several hours to reach full alertness, although the minutes shortly after waking are most problematic. Sleep inertia also interacts with both Process C and Process S, becoming worse and lasting longer when waking at the wrong circadian time in the middle of the night or from deep sleep.

Why you can feel sleepy after lunch but not sleepy before you go to bed

While alertness generally declines during the day, there is a window just before usual sleep time when it is difficult to fall asleep and alertness is relatively high. This 'wake maintenance zone' occurs because the circadian rhythm in alertness, which is still relatively high towards the end of the day, is not yet fully counteracted by the homeostatic increase for sleep building through the day. The end of this 'wake maintenance zone' coincides with the onset of production of the pineal hormone melatonin and is sometimes referred to as the opening of the 'sleep gate'. There is a rapid increase in sleepiness and ability to fall asleep at this time (Figure 6). Whether the onset of melatonin production causes this sleepiness, or is merely coincidental, is discussed later in this chapter.

The 'post-lunch dip' also results from a slight mismatch in the timing of Process S and Process C, and occurs regardless of whether food is consumed or not. This 'dip' in performance and alertness coincides with the usual crossing over of the rise in sleepiness due to Process S and the decrease in sleepiness due to Process C. If the two processes are slightly mismatched, then Process S will promote sleepiness before Process C has counteracted it, leading to a mid-afternoon lull. Not everyone experiences this dip, most likely due to small individual differences in the relative timing of the two processes. A larger mismatch between these processes, however, probably explains the habit of taking a siesta in some communities; shorter and later sleep at night leads to greater sleep pressure in the day which cannot be counteracted by the circadian rhythm in sleepiness, which has itself been shifted later by exposure to artificial light during the evening, facilitating a long nap in the afternoon. Add to that a heavy lunch and a few drinks, and your chances of staying awake are low!

Are you a lark or an owl? Morning types and evening types

If you are alert in the mornings and go to bed early, you are a 'lark', but if you hate mornings and want to keep going through the night, then you are an 'owl'. These terms have been used to try and describe the phenomenon of diurnal preference – whether you are a morning type or an evening type – based on the times when you prefer to sleep and when you do your best work. While you might think that this is a personal choice, diurnal preference is determined by the two-process model, and is partly encoded in your genes.

Imagine an experiment in which a group of people are kept on the same light–dark schedule (16 hours of light: 8 hours of dark) for several weeks: some people would go to bed and wake early; some would go to sleep late and lie-in; some would sleep for only 7 hours, some for 9 hours, and so on. Each person would find their own natural timing within the day – their diurnal preference, and their natural sleep timing and duration. Across a population, there would be a range of diurnal preferences and a range of sleep durations due to individual differences in how the circadian and homeostatic processes interact. For example, morning types, who tend to sleep and wake early, may have: i) a shorter-period circadian clock (close to or even less than 24 hours) that cycles faster than for evening types; ii) greater propensity to sleep early due to a quicker build-up or sensitivity to homeostatic sleep pressure; iii) greater propensity to wake early due to a quicker dissipation of homeostatic sleep pressure; or any combination of these factors.

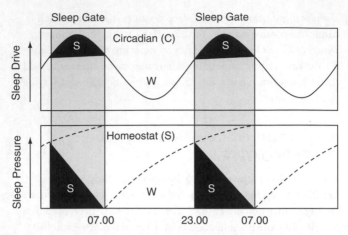

6. The two-process model of sleep regulation. A 24-hour circadian timer and a homeostatic driver (dotted line) interact to determine the timing, duration, and structure of sleep. A circadian-driven rhythm of sleep promotion during the night and arousal/wake during the day is opposed by a homeostatic driver which increasingly promotes sleep during the day. During sleep (shaded black), homeostatic sleep pressure is dissipated. The 'sleep gate' (shaded grey) occurs as a result of the combined effects of the circadian and homeostatic oscillators. During wake (W), sleep pressure rises but is opposed by Process C until sleep is initiated

Morning and evening types also differ in the time course of daytime sleepiness and performance, which is again determined by an interaction between Process C and Process S or the relative 'phase angle of entrainment' (timing) between when sleep occurs and when the circadian 'day' occurs. Morning types will wake at an earlier alarm-clock time – their sleep is advanced compared to evening types. Although their sleep rhythm is earlier, however, it tends not to be shifted quite as much as their internal circadian system, which means that morning types sleep and wake at a relatively later circadian phase than evening types. Morning types therefore wake later in their 'day', as it were, and consequently have high alertness and performance in the morning which declines rapidly through the day. Evening types, on the other hand, wake earlier in their circadian 'day' and are therefore more sleepy and poorer performers in the morning but do not decline as much as morning types by the end of the day. The behavioural differences reported by morning and evening types – that morning types feel more alert in the morning and prefer to perform critical tasks at this time, whereas evening types feel better and perform better later in the day, can therefore be explained by the circadian phase at which they wake. These differences are remarkably consistent despite all the factors that can affect daytime alertness patterns in the real world, such as the consumption of caffeinated drinks, work, stress, and so on, illustrating the critical role and relationship between Process C and Process S in determining daytime alertness, mood, and performance patterns.

Light, circadian rhythms, melatonin, sleep, and arousal

An important consideration in sleep–wake regulation is the role of light, exposure to which can affect both circadian timing (Process C) and sleepiness and performance directly (Process S). Light has a number of 'non-visual' effects on human physiology separate and apart from vision, including resetting the timing of the circadian pacemaker, acutely improving subjective and objective measures of alertness, increasing nighttime heart rate and core temperature levels, and affecting some hormones, including suppressing pineal melatonin production.

Light and sleep

The circadian clock in the suprachiasmatic nuclei (SCN) in the brain generates a rhythm that is near to, but not exactly, 24 hours, and in order to ensure that circadian rhythms are timed appropriately with the real world, environmental time cues must reset this internal clock every day. Under normal circumstances, exposure to the 24-hour pattern of light and dark synchronizes (entrains) biological rhythms to environmental rhythms (Figure 5). The 24-hour light–dark cycle is the most important environmental time signal, and this light information is captured exclusively by the eyes in mammals – eye loss abolishes photoentrainment. The SCN receives a direct projection from the eye via the retinohypothalamic tract (the nerve pathway from the retina to the hypothalamus), and light detected via the retina is therefore the primary '*Zeitgeber*' (time-giver) that synchronizes the timing of sleep and other circadian rhythms. In the entrained state, the multiple physiological and behavioural rhythms are appropriately phase- or time-locked to allow optimum function. Failure to receive this light–dark information, as experienced by most totally blind individuals, causes the circadian pacemaker to revert to its natural non-24-hour period and become desynchronized from the 24-hour day. Consequently, the majority of totally blind people suffer from a sleep disorder called 'non-24-hour sleep–wake disorder' as their sleep–wake cycle, alertness, and performance patterns and other rhythms become desynchronized from the 24-hour social day on which they attempt to live (see Chapter 6). Circadian misalignment also occurs in sighted subjects who are not exposed to a stable 24-hour light–dark cycle, for example in night shift-workers or after a rapid change in light–dark patterns following transmeridian travel ('jetlag'), causing serious sleep and health consequences (Chapter 9). Daily exposure to a stable 24-hour light–dark cycle is therefore required to maintain normal circadian entrainment and sleep timing.

Light also has a direct effect on Process S in that light exposure can acutely enhance alertness and performance during both the day and the night and affect the depth of subsequent nighttime sleep. Brain imaging following light exposure shows increased activity in many of the brain areas involved in alertness, cognition, and memory (thalamus, hippocampus, brainstem) and mood (amygdala). Inappropriately timed light exposure can therefore disrupt not only sleep and circadian timing but also levels of alertness, performance, and mood.

Rhythm and blues

Our understanding of how light regulates sleep and circadian rhythms has been revolutionized over the past few years with the discovery of an entirely new photoreceptor system in the mammalian eye, including that of humans. This novel photoreceptor is not located in the part of the eye containing the rods (night vision) and cones (day vision) that are used to generate an image of the world, but in the ganglion cells whose projections form the optic nerve. The ganglion cells of the retina provide the functional connection between the eye and the brain, but a small number of specialized ganglion cells (1–3%) are directly light-sensitive and project to parts of the brain involved in sleep and circadian rhythm control, including the SCN and another hypothalamic area called the ventrolateral preoptic area (VLPO; see Chapter 3).

These photosensitive retinal ganglion cells (pRGCs) contain a light-sensitive pigment called melanopsin (also called Opn4). Note that melanopsin should not be confused with the pineal hormone melatonin, or the skin pigment melanin – all are completely different! Melanopsin is most sensitive to visible short-wavelength 'blue light' with a peak sensitivity to light with a wavelength of about 480 nanometres. This system still works to shift the circadian clock or regulate sleep even in animals or people in whom the rods and cones used for vision are completely abolished and who are otherwise totally visually blind. As long as the ganglion cell layer of the eye is intact, entrainment can still occur. This fact raises important implications for ophthalmologists, who are largely unaware of this new photoreceptor system and its impact on human physiology. For example, where the pRGC system is still intact, individuals should be encouraged (where possible) to expose their eyes to sufficient daytime light to maintain normal circadian entrainment and sleep–wake timing. Blind patients who are scheduled to have their eyes removed for non-essential reasons should be assessed to determine whether their eyes are still functioning to detect light and synchronize the circadian system, as bilateral eye loss will result in development of non-24-hour sleep–wake disorder. Furthermore, patients with diseases of the inner retina which result in retinal ganglion cell death, such as glaucoma, are at particular risk of circadian rhythm and sleep disruption. Such individuals should receive counselling regarding the problems of sleep disruption and would be strong candidates for treatment with appropriately timed melatonin, which has been shown to consolidate sleep timing in totally blind patients (see Chapter 6).

Blue-light-detecting pRGCs not only shift the timing of the circadian clock, but play a major role in suppressing melatonin production, reducing sleepiness, improving reaction times, and activating areas of the brain mediating alertness and sleep. These effects of light have widespread clinical and occupational applications in treating sleep disorders and fatigue associated with circadian rhythm disorders, depression, dementia, and cancer, or anywhere where a sleepiness countermeasure would be beneficial, for example in schools, colleges, and offices, 24/7 professions such as nursing, the police, and firefighters, and other safety-sensitive occupations including pilots, the military, control centres, power plants, and so on (see Chapter 9). Blue-light therapy in the morning has also been shown to be effective in the treatment of seasonal affective disorder ('winter depression'), which is caused by seasonal changes in light–dark exposure.

The timing of light exposure is also particularly important. Light can either phase advance the clock, shifting behaviour and metabolism to an earlier time, or phase delay the circadian system depending on the timing of exposure. Under normal conditions, light around dusk and the first part of the night (18:00 to 6:00 hours) causes a phase delay of the clock, whereas light exposure in the late night and around dawn (6:00 to 18:00 hours) will phase advance the clock. The relationship between the timing of a stimulus and the direction and magnitude of the resultant shift is described in a phase response curve (PRC), which is critical when considering the effects of altered light–dark exposure experienced during jetlag or during shift-work (Chapter 9). Although not as sensitive as the visual system, circadian rhythms and alertness can still be affected by relatively low light levels, if exposure is over several hours. Under these circumstances, relatively dim indoor room light from bedside lamps and computer screens has measurable effects on the clock and sleep systems, and may exacerbate sleep disorders (Chapter 6).

The 'Dracula' hormone – melatonin and sleep

The pRGCs tell the body when it is light, but how does the body know when it is dark? The 'Dracula' hormone melatonin provides this signal as it is released only at night and production is inhibited by light. Pineal melatonin is the major biochemical correlate of darkness and provides an internal representation of the environmental night-length. As night-length changes with the seasons in non-equatorial latitudes, melatonin not only encodes the daily night-length but also the time of year (season).

Melatonin is synthesized from tryptophan, a dietary amino acid, which is converted over several steps to serotonin and then melatonin. It is produced mainly by the pineal gland, although the retina and other regions of the body may produce small amounts which are thought to help with local timekeeping. Levels peak in plasma and saliva at approximately 2 a.m. under normal conditions, with its major urinary metabolite (6-sulphatoxymelatonin) peaking around 4:30 a.m. Pineal cells produce melatonin 'upon request' from the biological clock – it is not stored and is secreted by the pineal gland under the direct control of the SCN. Unusually, the pathway from the SCN proceeds via the spinal cord (via the superior cervical ganglion, or SCG) before returning to the pineal gland, which means that tetraplegic individuals with spinal damage at the upper cervical level have no melatonin production (although other circadian rhythms not requiring this pathway, for example the cortisol, temperature, and sleep–wake rhythms, are relatively normal).

Light exposure exclusively to the eyes at night inhibits melatonin production acutely and provides an indirect assessment of light input to the SCN via the eye–SCN–pineal pathway. There are melatonin receptors on SCN neurones, and melatonin is thought to provide feedback to the clock to ensure proper synchronization of internal rhythms. Given the close temporal relationship between the SCN and melatonin production, the melatonin rhythm is often used as a 'phase-marker' of the circadian clock in human studies.

The direct role of melatonin on sleep is less clear, however. While melatonin production coincides with sleep in diurnal animals such as humans, nocturnal animals such as rats and hamsters also produce melatonin at night, during their active episode, and many mice strains do not produce any melatonin at all, suggesting that melatonin may not have any effect on sleep. Certainly, the circadian sleep propensity rhythm in humans is closely correlated with the melatonin profile – the opening of the 'sleep gate' occurs simultaneously with the onset of melatonin. These events may simply be contemporaneous, however, as individuals who do not produce melatonin (for example, tetraplegic individuals, many people taking beta-blockers, pinealectomized patients) still exhibit circadian sleep–wake rhythms and have only minor changes in sleep structure. The circadian system, rather than melatonin itself, therefore probably opens the gate for sleep and switches on melatonin at the same time.

Another association between melatonin and sleepiness is the fact that when melatonin is suppressed by light exposure at night, alertness levels also simultaneously improve. Light exposure in the daytime will also improve alertness, however, at a time when melatonin is not produced, suggesting that either melatonin is not a direct mediator of alertness and/or separate mechanisms exist during the day and night for enhancement of alertness by light. Taking synthetic melatonin will also have a mild sleepiness-inducing effect especially when no natural melatonin is being released which, when coupled with its ability to shift the timing of the clock, makes melatonin useful in treating sleep disorders associated with circadian rhythm disruption such as shift-work, jetlag, non-24-hour rhythms in the blind, and advanced and delayed sleep phase disorders (see Chapter 6) if timed appropriately.

What happens without any sleep?

Understanding the role of sleep and circadian rhythms on physiology and metabolism requires carefully controlled laboratory experiments. A simple approach to examine the direct effect of sleep is to compare what happens when subjects are allowed to sleep versus what happens if they are made to stay awake all night. Such sleep deprivation studies have demonstrated that many hormones and peptides are influenced by the circadian system, sleep, or a combination of both. Pineal melatonin levels are virtually the same whether sleep occurs or not, although it is strongly suppressed if the lights are not very dim. Cortisol, a hormone produced by the adrenal glands, is also relatively unchanged whether asleep or awake, rising during the night to a maximum shortly before we usually wake (even if not asleep), although waking from sleep causes a small additional elevation. Conversely, some hormones, for example growth hormone (GH), are very strongly sleep-dependent with little influence of the circadian system. GH is secreted primarily during slow-wave sleep (SWS), and there are very low levels under conditions of sleep deprivation. Thyroid-stimulating hormone (TSH) has a small peak close to sleep onset under normal conditions and appears to be under minimal circadian control. When measured without sleep, however, a robust circadian rhythm in TSH is revealed, with a night-time peak which is usually suppressed by sleep at night. So going without sleep will decrease GH levels and elevate TSH.

Not getting enough sleep?

We are only beginning to understand what happens if you don't get enough sleep every night and suffer from chronic sleep deficiency. Most of the work to date has concentrated on the effects of sleep deficiency on alertness and performance, but emerging data also show serious consequences on metabolism and health (see Chapter 7). Under ideal conditions, the sleep pressure accumulated during wakefulness is dissipated during sleep to the extent that alertness is restored to near-maximal levels upon wakening. Several lines of evidence suggest that young adults would sleep about 8.5 hours per night if given sufficient opportunity, and older adults about 7.5 hours, much more than is usually experienced by most people. Failure to achieve an appropriate amount of sleep leads to chronic sleep deficiency, or the accumulation of a 'sleep debt'. Like many monetary contracts, however, there are strict rules on when this sleep debt must be repaid, and it cannot be put off indefinitely without incurring large penalties, in this case on health. Unlike most monetary contracts, however, sleep deficiency has to be repaid each day and sleeping in at weekends does not seem to be sufficient to repay a week's worth of bad sleep. Unfortunately, sleep credits are very difficult to obtain, although getting extra sleep shortly before an anticipated episode of sleep deprivation can be helpful. Simply put, regular (daily), substantial sleep deposits are needed to maintain a healthy balance in the sleep bank.

The detrimental effects of chronic sleep loss can quickly become as severe as acute deprivation. After about 2 weeks with fewer than 6 hours of sleep per night, performance levels fall to the same level as someone with 24 hours of acute sleep deprivation; with 4 hours in bed per night, it takes only 7 days to reach that level, and after 2 weeks, performance is equivalent to 2–3 days without sleep. Worryingly, self-assessed ratings of sleepiness do not change at the same rate, suggesting that we cannot accurately judge how impaired we are when sleep deprived, rather like when we think we can be great drivers after drinking too much. If acute and chronic sleep deprivation are combined, for example by failing to get enough recovery sleep after staying up all night on repeated occasions, the harmful effects on performance are

Box 2: Sleep deprivation and torture

Sleep deprivation, or 'sleep management', has recently come to the fore through its use as an enhanced interrogation technique. Sleep deprivation for up to 180 hours – 7.5 days – is at the time of writing permitted by the US government, having previously been deemed illegal. It is generally achieved using loud noise and shackles to maintain an extremely uncomfortable posture that makes it virtually impossible to sleep. Under US regulations, only 8 hours of sleep are required after this 7.5-day sleep deprivation before a further 7.5 days can be imposed. Imagine similar restrictions for food or water. Such sleep deprivation is used to affect psychological state, although the myriad effects of sleep deprivation on metabolism and immune function are also likely to be damaging. Sleep deprivation causes a number of neurobiological effects including deterioration in reaction time, memory, and cognitive abilities. It quite quickly causes subjects to have 'hypnogogic hallucinations', changes in perception that represent visualization of dreams or other images due to incursion of REM brain activity patterns into wakefulness. More serious events include impairment of emotional processing and ultimately psychosis.

As sleep deprivation decreases pain thresholds and increases hunger, it is also thought to enhance other interrogation techniques, such as dietary manipulation. Even though medical supervision is required, doctors receive little or no training in sleep medicine and have no experience in identifying the short- or long-term consequences of acute or chronic sleep deprivation. Society often trivializes sleep deprivation and, consequently, its full impact as an interrogation technique is not appreciated. It is important to remember that sleep is an essential behaviour, as important as nutrition in terms of survival. The 1975 UN Convention Against Torture provides 'Protection of all persons from being subjected to torture and other cruel, inhuman or degrading treatment or punishment'. Clearly, prolonged sleep deprivation breaches these requirements.

multiplied up to 10-times. It is not yet known how many nights of extended sleep are needed to reverse this decline, although the occasional lie-in at the weekend is probably not going to be enough. Just like going to the gym or following a diet plan, it takes a concerted effort every day to get enough sleep and avoid the health and safety effects of acute and chronic sleep deprivation.

Chapter 3
The sleeping brain

As outlined in Chapter 2, sleep is a highly complex state that arises from two broadly opposing mechanisms involving both the 24-hour body clock (circadian system; Process C) and a wake-dependent homeostatic build-up of sleep pressure (Process S) (Figure 6). These drivers coordinate REM and NREM sleep and the activity of multiple brain regions, neurotransmitters, and modulatory hormones, none of which are exclusive to the generation of sleep (Figure 7). This huge complexity explains why disentangling the neuroscience of sleep has been so difficult, and probably explains why sleep patterns are so variable between humans and across species. Sleep structure, like an individual's personality, is the product of diverse environmental stimuli and dynamic endogenous interactions. Here we review the major brain structures and neurotransmitter systems involved in the generation of sleep in mammals. This is not an easy chapter, so you may want to go and get a cup of coffee before you read on!

The suprachiasmatic nuclei (SCN) and the molecular clock

The destruction (lesioning) of small areas of the rat brain, and specifically the frontal part of the hypothalamus, identified a small paired cluster of around 20,000 cells known as the

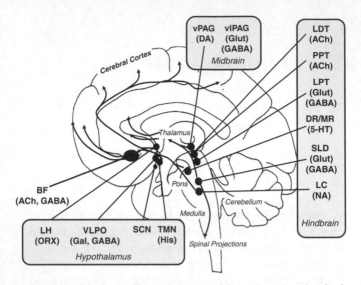

7. **Diagram of the brain, illustrating some of the main regions involved in sleep–wake regulation. The brain structures and their associated key neurotransmitters are shown.** *Abbreviations for brain regions*: **BF** = basal forebrain; **DR/MR** = dorsal/medial raphe nucleus; **LC** = locus coeruleus; **LDT** = laterodorsal tegmental nuclei; **LH** = lateral hypothalamus; **LPT** = lateral pontine tegmentum; **PPT** = pedunculopontine tegmental nuclei; **SCN** = suprachiasmatic nuclei; **SLD** = sublaterodorsal nucleus; **TMN** = tuberomammillary nucleus; **VLPO** = ventrolateral preoptic nuclei; **vPAG** = ventral periaqueductal grey; **vlPAG** = ventrolateral periaqueductal grey. *Abbreviations for neurotransmitters*: **5-HT** = serotonin; **ACh** = acetylcholine; **DA** = dopamine; **GABA** = γ-aminobutyric acid; **Gal** = galanin; **Glut** = glutamate; **His** = histamine; **NA** = noradrenaline; **ORX** = orexin

suprachiasmatic nuclei (SCN) as critical elements in organizing 24-hour rhythms of behaviour such as drinking and locomotion. Further proof that the SCN contains the 'master circadian clock' came from studies in the 1980s and 1990s showing that the effects of SCN lesions could be reversed by transplanting SCN tissue from one animal to another, which restored many 24-hour rhythms, including the sleep–wake cycle.

Each cell in the SCN is also a separate clock; individual SCN neurones show near-24-hour rhythms of activity and somehow co-coordinate their individual electrical activity to give the overall near-24-hour rhythmic output from the SCN. The demonstration that isolated SCN neurones can generate near-24-hour oscillations showed that the mechanism that makes the clock 'tick' must be a subcellular molecular mechanism. From the 1970s, the results from research on the fruit fly (*Drosophila*), mutant mice, and mutant hamsters, combined with inspired guess-work and simple good luck, led to the generation of a molecular model for circadian rhythm generation that depends upon the activity of a group of critical 'clock genes'. At the core is a molecular feedback loop whereby the proteins BMAL1 and CLOCK act as regulators of gene transcription and control the production of *Per1*, *Per2*, *Per3*, *Cry1*, and *Cry2* proteins. In brief, the CLOCK:BMAL1 proteins bind to regions of the *period* and *cryptochrome* genes, driving *Per* and *Cry* protein expression. The PER proteins then interact with CRY proteins to form a protein complex in the cell cytoplasm. This protein complex then enters the cell nucleus and drives a negative feedback loop by inhibiting CLOCK:BMAL1-mediated transcription, effectively switching off production of PER and CRY. The PER/CRY complex is then degraded, the inhibition of CLOCK:BMAL1-mediated transcription is lifted, and CLOCK:BMAL1 is once more free to drive transcription. This molecular of protein production and degradation takes about 24 hours to complete.

Such molecular clocks are not confined to SCN cells; it is now clear that most cells of the body possess the ability to generate a circadian oscillation independently of the SCN (albeit damped and not self-sustaining). This finding transformed the view of the mammalian circadian system. The assumption was that the SCN forced 24-hour rhythmicity on the rest of the body, whereas we now appreciate that there is a more hierarchal arrangement of multiple peripheral clocks, synchronized by the 'master' SCN, or the 'conductor' of the rhythmic orchestra, using both chemical and neuronal signals. The circadian system in turn receives multiple feedbacks from the body and a variety of organ systems, with the net result being a complex arrangement of reciprocal interactions all contributing to the period, phase, and amplitude of an individual's circadian rhythms. The uniqueness of the SCN, however, is that it coordinates the clocks in other tissues and it alone is the only part of the brain able to restore rhythmicity when transplanted into an SCN-lesioned host.

This molecular oscillation within the SCN is aligned to the light–dark cycle detected by the eye. The retinohypothalamic tract projecting to the SCN releases the neurotransmitters glutamate and pituitary adenylate cyclase-activating polypeptide (PACAP). Several intracellular signalling cascades are then activated which ultimately lead to the up-regulation of *Per1* and *Per2* genes. The subsequent synthesis of PER1 and PER2 proteins results in prolonged suppression of CLOCK/BMAL1 activity. It is this light-induced suppression of CLOCK/BMAL1 transcriptional drive that appears critical for entrainment of the molecular clock to the local light cycle.

While light is the primary environmental time cue for resetting the SCN, it is important to stress that a number of different entrainment pathways are emerging that have been shown to adjust peripheral clocks in the liver, gut, and other organs independently of the SCN. Indeed, lack of internal synchrony between the different organ systems appears to cause many of the symptoms of jetlag. The peripheral clocks receive conflicting timing cues from the SCN (which is itself in the process of adjustment), and from the environment by irregular sleep-activity schedules (Process S), abnormal light exposure, and food intake. Thus the normal alignment of internal physiological and metabolic processes is lost, with potential health consequences (Chapters 7, 8, and 9).

The homeostatic drivers

Sleep is also homeostatically regulated (Process S) such that the pressure to sleep increases with increasing time awake, and dissipates during subsequent sleep. Sleep deprivation drives a compensatory increase in the intensity of sleep, as measured by NREM slow-wave activity, and the duration of recovery sleep. Although the dynamics of homeostatic sleep regulation have been studied extensively, relatively little is understood about the nature of this process. In contrast to the clear anatomical location of the circadian master clock within the SCN, the homeostatic sleep 'nuclei' and the regulatory substances driving sleep propensity remain poorly understood.

Studies a century ago showed that cerebrospinal fluid (CSF) contained a substance that accumulated during wakefulness and could induce sleep when transferred from a sleep-deprived donor to another animal. The hunt for 'the' homeostatic sleep driver has centred upon the concept of a sleep factor which fulfils all or some of the following criteria: (i) if the agent is introduced into the brain, it will enhance sleep; (ii) if the agent is blocked, sleep will be reduced; (iii) the agent should vary with sleep drive or sleep propensity; (iv) the agent should act on brain circuits known to be involved in sleep; (v) the agent may be altered in pathological states associated with sleep.

On the basis of these criteria, many substances have now been implicated. For example, interleukin-1β (IL-1β), tumour necrosis factor-α (TNF-α), growth hormone-releasing hormone (GHRH), prostaglandin D_2, and adenosine have all been linked to the regulation of NREM sleep. For the regulation of REM sleep, prolactin, nitric oxide (NO), and vasoactive intestinal polypeptide (VIP) have been similarly implicated. By way of example, the evidence for adenosine regulation of NREM sleep can be summarized as follows.

The sleep-inducing effects of adenosine were first shown in cats during the 1950s. The adenosine receptor antagonists (adenosine blockers) caffeine and theophylline, found in coffee and tea, are widely used as stimulants of the central nervous system to induce vigilance and increase the time spent awake. Caffeine reduces slow-wave EEG activity in the following sleep episode, and caffeine consumption during prolonged wakefulness counteracts the typical effects of sleep deprivation on the waking and sleep EEG.

Adenosine is a by-product of energy metabolism and ATP utilization. Extracellular adenosine concentrations have been shown to increase in the brain with increased metabolism, neural activity, and wakefulness. Measurements of adenosine in the brains of freely moving cats and rats across the sleep–wake cycle show significantly lower levels of adenosine in the basal forebrain during sleep than during wakefulness.

It is important to stress that adenosine is not the only potential sleep regulatory substance. A variety of sleep regulatory agents can act to differentially promote sleep and change the electrical activity of neurones in very specific regions of the brain associated with sleep regulation (Figure 7). Adenosine acts on basal forebrain neurones to promote sleep; by contrast, GHRH, TNF, and IL1 act on anterior hypothalamic neurones to promote NREM; TNF and IL1 also act on the locus coeruleus; and IL1 acts on the dorsal raphe to promote sleep. Such results all suggest that the search for a single 'holy grail' sleep substance for a single homeostatic driver is going to be a futile exercise.

Brain regions and the neurotransmitters of sleep and wakefulness

The circadian and homeostatic processes regulate multiple brain circuits and neurotransmitter systems. Wakefulness involves the

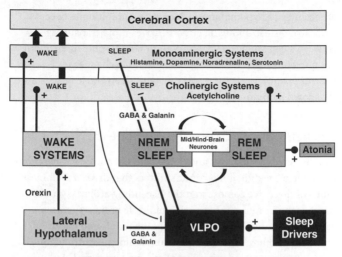

8. The major brain structures and neurotransmitters involved in driving the sleep–wake cycle. During the wake state, orexin neurones within the lateral hypothalamus project to and excite the monoaminergic and cholinergic neurones. Collectively, these neurotransmitters drive wakefulness throughout the brain and consciousness in the cerebral cortex. Also during wakefulness, the monoaminergic neurones inhibit the ventrolateral preoptic nuclei (VLPO). During sleep, circadian and homeostatic sleep drivers activate the VLPO, which releases GABA and galanin to inhibit the orexin neurones within the lateral hypothalamus and inhibit the monoaminergic and cholinergic neurones. The flip/flop every 70–90 minutes between NREM and REM sleep is driven by neurones in the mid- and hind-brain. During REM sleep, monoaminergic neurones remain inhibited, but cholinergic neurones are activated. REM-on neurones project to the spinal cord and drive muscle paralysis (**atonia**)

activation of neuronal clusters within the brainstem, hypothalamus, and basal forebrain which in turn promote arousal within the thalamus and cerebral cortex (Figure 7). Sleep induction is driven by a rapid reduction in arousal, which has been linked to an inhibitory switch controlled by GABA/galanin-containing neurones in the ventrolateral preoptic region (VLPO) of the anterior hypothalamus. Reciprocal inhibition between arousal and sleep-inducing circuits drives rapid transitions between sleep and wake states. A summary of some of the main brain regions involved in sleep-wake and the changes in neurotransmitter release associated with sleep and arousal states are shown in Figure 8.

The neurotransmitters of wakefulness

As illustrated in Figures 7 and 8, the cerebral cortex of the brain is bathed in a cocktail of neurotransmitters that drive wakefulness. Much of this drive comes from the 'ascending arousal system', which is the term used to describe multiple brain structures within the brainstem, thalamus, hypothalamus, and basal forebrain which release multiple monoamine neurotransmitters (histamine, dopamine, noradrenaline, serotonin) and a cholinergic neurotransmitter (acetylcholine) all of which drive wakefulness. The ascending arousal system is itself activated during wakefulness by direct projections from orexin-producing neurones in the lateral hypothalamus. Destruction of orexinergic neurones has been shown to cause some forms of narcolepsy. Also during wakefulness the VLPO is inhibited by multiple inputs from the monoaminergic systems and other brain areas, including the hypothalamus.

The generation of NREM and REM sleep

As illustrated in Figure 8, activation of the VLPO by sleep drivers (circadian and homeostatic) triggers both NREM and REM sleep. It does this by inhibiting the orexin neurones within the lateral hypothalamus. The VLPO also inhibits directly both the monoaminergic and cholinergic systems during NREM (Figure 8). During REM, the monoaminergic system remains inhibited, but the cholinergic system is activated by REM-on neurones within the mid-brain. A key sleep driver is adenosine, which is thought to accumulate in the extracellular spaces of the basal forebrain which activates the VLPO by several indirect and direct pathways.

The NREM-REM flip-flop

The cycle of NREM and REM sleep arises from neurones in the mid- and hind-brain (Figure 8). The REM-off neurones are located within the ventrolateral periaqueductal grey (vlPAG) of the mid-brain and the lateral pontine tegmentum (LPT) of the hind-brain (Figure 7). Damage to these regions greatly increases the amount of REM sleep, suggesting that they normally inhibit REM sleep. The REM-on neurones are located within the sublaterodorsal nucleus (SLD) of the hind-brain (Figure 7) which is active during REM sleep. Damage to the SLD greatly reduces REM and muscle paralysis (atonia); indeed, individuals may walk around during sleep. The 'flip-flop' between NREM and REM sleep involves inhibitory interactions between neurones within the REM-on and REM-off neuronal centres. The REM-on SLD also contains neurones that project directly to the spinal cord and produce muscle atonia. Yet another projection from the SLD goes to the basal forebrain and PPT/LDT (Figure 7) and produces the EEG components of REM sleep. Clifford Saper's laboratory at Harvard has done much to provide our understanding of this 'flip-flop switch' controlling sleep.

Multiple sleep genes and multiple patterns of sleep-wake

In the 1930s, studies showed that monozygotic twins, who share 100% of their genes, had more similar sleep times and sleep durations compared to dizygotic twins, who share only 50% of their genes. More recent studies in both humans and mice have shown that patterns of NREM and REM sleep architecture show greater levels of similarity in closely related individuals. That sleep has a genetic component is perhaps not too surprising – but which genes are involved?

There is now good evidence linking specific changes in clock genes with morningness and eveningness. For example, polymorphisms of the human *Per 1–3* genes are associated with extreme morning types ('larks'). Morning preference is also associated with mutations in the kinases (*CK1* delta and *CK1* epsilon) that phosphorylate PER proteins leading to abnormalities in PER protein stability and movement into the nucleus. In mice, mutations in *CRY1* will advance sleep, whilst mutations in *CRY2* and *CLOCK* will delay sleep.

Clock genes have also been linked to the homeostatic regulation of sleep. Mice with mutations in the *CLOCK* gene sleep around 2 hours less than non-mutant mice, whilst mice with mutations in both *CRY1* and *CRY2* show longer sleep episodes. Studies by Paul Franken and colleagues have shown that *Per1* and *Per2* levels in the forebrain of mice increase with sleep deprivation and decrease during sleep recovery. The mechanisms through which these genes regulate sleep remain a mystery.

In view of the involvement of so many neurotransmitters in the generation of sleep (Figure 7), we would predict that mutations in the genes involved in the production of these neurotransmitters and their receptors, modulators, and ion channels will be associated with sleep and sleep abnormalities, and this prediction – where tested – has been correct. Narcolepsy is perhaps the best example. Narcolepsy is a sleep disorder whereby individuals experience fragmented sleep, excessive daytime sleepiness, and abnormal REM sleep including cataplexy (a sudden loss of muscle tone), and it is a condition that has been linked to defects in the orexin (also called hypocretin) pathway (Figure 8). Drug manipulation, mutations in key genes, or targeted genetic disruption of the cholinergic system and monoaminergic system all disrupt the wake-promoting action of these neurotransmitters and their receptors (Figure 8). For example, histamine decarboxylase receptor knockout mice show increased REM sleep and wake fragmentation. These mice are also unable to remain awake for long episodes and show a behaviour very similar to narcolepsy.

At this time, it appears unlikely that there is a unique sleep neurotransmitter or brain structure – sleep and wakefulness seem to arise from a network of brain activity. During sleep, each person activates this network in a slightly different way, integrating daily experiences and past emotions, and accommodating the ageing process. Teasing apart, the dynamics of these endogenous and environmental contributions to both normal and abnormal sleep are going to keep neuroscientists busy for very many years to come.

Chapter 4
The reasons for sleep

The reasons why we sleep remain frustratingly unresolved. Many explanations have been proposed, but no one overarching hypothesis has emerged to explain why this major aspect of our behaviour exists. As discussed in Chapters 2 and 3, our explanation for how we sleep is fairly advanced, but this has not really helped us understand the 'why' or the evolutionary purpose of sleep. Here we ask two closely related questions: Do all animals sleep, and, if they do, why?

Do all animals sleep?

Most life, including unicellular organisms, shows daily 24-hour cycles of activity and rest. These 24-hour rhythms are driven by some form of endogenous circadian timer. Such a timer exists to fine-tune physiology and behaviour to anticipate the varying demands of the day–night cycle (external synchronization) and to ensure that the multiple internal rhythms are appropriately aligned (internal synchronization). The assumption by many has been that periods of inactivity represent 'sleep' and that the function of this inactivity is broadly conserved across all animals. Sleep researchers are markedly divided on this point, however.

Before we consider why animals might sleep, let us consider whether we can recognize a sleep-like state across the animal kingdom. The

Table 1. Behavioural criteria used to define sleep

1	A rapidly reversible state of immobility with greatly reduced sensory responsiveness. The rapid reversibility distinguishes sleep from coma or hibernation.
2	Increased arousal thresholds (requires more noise to be woken) and a decreased responsiveness to external stimulation.
3	Species-specific posture and place preference.
4	Behavioural rituals before sleep (e.g. circling, yawning, nest-making).
5	Circadian regulation and persistence of a ~24-hour rhythm under constant conditions.
6	A behaviour that is homeostatically regulated such that lost sleep is associated with an increased drive for sleep, with subsequent 'sleep rebound'.

definition of sleep in humans is based largely upon electroencephalography (EEG) (Chapter 2), but in the absence of a complex brain capable of generating a NREM-REM EEG, sleep has been more difficult to define. As a result, sleep researchers, and notably Irene Tobler, have developed a series of non-EEG behavioural criteria to try and help define sleep, summarized in Table 1. Of these six behaviours, sleep rebound has been regarded as particularly important. Using both EEG-defined sleep states (Chapter 2) and the behavioural criteria outlined in Table 1, let us now consider the possible existence of sleep across the animal world.

Mammals

All mammals show some form of sleep. When mammals are sleep-deprived, they show sleep rebound. In humans, a reduction in sleep will drive extended sleep the following night with increased amounts of slow-wave sleep. Of the few other groups of terrestrial mammals studied in any detail (e.g. rodents, cats, dogs, monkeys), sleep can be defined on the basis of both behavioural criteria (Table 1) and NREM (high-amplitude, low-frequency) and REM (low-amplitude, high-frequency) EEG patterns (see Chapter 2). REM-like sleep and the accompanying muscle atonia has been shown in all mammals, including the egg-laying platypus which exhibits REM sleep for more than 60% of the total sleep time. Special forms of sleep have been described in marine mammals. In fur seals, the EEG on land is similar to most other terrestrial mammals; both eyes are closed, there are cycles of NREM-REM activity, and the EEG is synchronized across the left and right sides of the brain. In water, however, sleep is often unihemispheric (one-sided), with a sleep EEG on one side of the brain, with the opposite eye closed and an inactive flipper. Thus one half of the body appears to be asleep whilst the other is awake. Fully marine mammals such as the whales and dolphins also show unihemispheric sleep, but in contrast to the fur seals have never been reported to show sleep across both the left and right sides of the brain simultaneously. This remarkable property of the sleeping brain seems to allow marine mammals to swim continuously. As a result, the marine mammals provide an important exception to the behavioural criteria that define sleep in Table 1.

Birds

In broad terms, birds resemble mammals in their sleep EEG. Birds show both REM and NREM EEG patterns during their inactive periods which are accompanied by specific sleep postures. Bird REM is also associated with rapid eye movements with reduced muscle tone, although not the complete atonia seen in mammals. Episodes of REM in birds are typically very much shorter (less than 10 seconds) compared to mammals, and overall birds spend less time in REM sleep. The original explanation for shortened REM was that it protects birds from falling out of trees when asleep by minimizing the muscle atonia associated with REM! This now seems unlikely, as perching birds utilize tendons to lock onto branches rather than sustained muscle contraction, and very short REM episodes are seen in birds such as geese that sleep on the ground. Recently, the suggestion has been that birds do in fact show long REM but at the level of the brainstem, not at the level of the cortex. The behavioural criteria for sleep are also broadly fulfilled in birds (Table 1), although there are differences compared to mammals. For example, birds seem to lack REM sleep rebound following sleep disruption. In migratory birds, both EEG and behaviourally defined sleep are reduced by 70% compared to levels of sleep when not migrating, and this is not followed by any obvious reduction in cognitive behaviour or sleep rebound.

It is worth noting that birds, along with reptiles, amphibians, and fish, have in addition to their SCN, circadian clocks within the eyes and pineal gland that contribute to the generation of 24-hour rhythms in behaviour. These clocks are in turn regulated by extra-retinal photoreceptors within the pineal gland, hypothalamus, and forebrain. Remarkably, sunlight can pass through the skin, feathers, scales, skull, and brain tissue, and although it is scattered and absorbed, there is sufficient light left for the photoreceptors within the brain to gain an overall assessment of the amount of light within the environment and hence time of day.

Reptiles and amphibians

There have been relatively few studies on amphibian and reptile sleep. From the 1960s, sleep-like states (Table 1) have been described in frogs and toads, which show stereotypical sleep behaviours, increased arousal thresholds, and what has been suggested by some researchers to be an NREM sleep-like EEG with increased amplitude and reduced frequency. The few studies on reptiles show elements of behavioural sleep (Table 1); for example, tortoises and marine turtles show rest periods that are accompanied by decreased sensitivity to stimuli, and there is good evidence for rebound sleep after rest disruption. Some reptiles (e.g. lizards and some crocodilians) are reported to show a slow NREM-like EEG during the resting state. By contrast, tortoises, turtles, and other crocodilians appear to lack this NREM-like EEG. There is some evidence for an REM-like EEG sleep pattern in reptiles, particularly lizards, and some species show distinctive eye and head movements that have been suggested to represent an REM sleep state. In general, however, there is weak evidence for REM sleep in reptiles.

Fish

Many teleost (bony) fish appear to show behavioural sleep-like states both in the wild and under laboratory conditions. In the laboratory, and occasionally demonstrated in the field, nocturnal rest in many species is accompanied by reduced respiration and raised response thresholds. Many fish also appear to adopt sleep-specific postures. For example, members of the Wrasse family (*Labridae*) lie on the sand on their sides during the night, and often in groups, whilst many species partially bury themselves. Some ocean species will float in open water. A frequently adopted position is to float with the head slightly raised compared to the tail. Reef fish retreat into small holes within the coral during the rest phase, and the timing of this retreat is remarkably precise. These precisely timed rest–activity cycles suggest the involvement of a circadian timer. Zebrafish (*Danio rerio*) and several other species, such as perch (*Cichlosoma* species) have been shown to respond to rest disruption with extended 'sleep' the next day, suggesting the presence of homeostatic sleep rebound recovery processes. There has been no demonstration of NREM or REM sleep in fish, although periods of eye movement during sleep/rest have been likened to REM.

Invertebrates

Invertebrates make up 98% of animal species, yet sleep remains poorly understood in these taxa. A significant number of invertebrate species show sleep-like states (Table 1). In the cephalopods (squids and octopi), increased arousal thresholds are accompanied by both a narrowing of pupils and colour changes. Insects and other arthropods such as scorpions show periods of reduced sensory responsiveness over the 24-hour day. Honey bees show increased responsiveness to visual stimuli during the day which is depressed at night, when they also exhibit specific body, head, and antennae postures, as do cockroaches. There is also evidence of sleep rebound in bees; 12 hours of sleep deprivation during the night causes an increase of antennae immobility and 'sleep' posture during the following night.

The fruit fly *Drosophila* is the current model of choice to try and understand the biology of sleep. *Drosophila* has a well-characterized and easy-to-manipulate genome, there are multiple well-archived mutants, flies possess a similar neurotransmitter system to the vertebrates, they are cheap to maintain, and have fast breeding cycles. Flies show a typical posture during behavioural rest, with elevated arousal thresholds. They also show clear sleep rebound in response to sleep deprivation. Stimulants such as caffeine cause a dose-dependent decrease in normal resting behaviour, whilst antihistamines increase the amount of resting behaviour. Also, flies that lack the critical circadian clock gene (*period*) (see Chapter 3) still show sleep rebound in response to sleep deprivation, suggesting that sleep and circadian cycles are not one and the same.

This brief summary suggests that sleep in some form probably exists across the animal kingdom but this view is not universal. A critical examination of the literature by Jerome Siegal led him to conclude that very few animals display all the behavioural criteria for sleep – few really show both a decreased level of arousal or rest rebound after deprivation. Other researchers argue that sleep should be defined on the basis of EEG alone. Using these criteria, invertebrates do not sleep at all, and the vertebrates fall into four broad categories: (i) species that rest but do not show a clear sleep EEG (fish and amphibians); (ii) species that show NREM sleep only (most reptiles); (iii) species showing NREM and partial REM or short episodes of REM (some reptiles and birds); (iv) species showing robust cycles of REM and NREM sleep (mammals). This lack of a consensus regarding a definition of sleep, and by extension the presence or absence of sleep across the animal kingdom, highlights the key problem in trying to address the evolutionary function of sleep. How can we determine the evolutionary function of sleep if we can't even decide what sleep is?

Variation in sleep duration across the mammals

The duration of sleep varies strikingly across the small proportion of mammalian species measured (Table 2) and has led to the suggestion that if this variation can be linked to a particular ecology or physiological capability, then an explanation for why sleep exists could be deduced. In mammals, there are some general trends. Overall, sleep times decrease with increased body size. Also, predatory species tend to have more sleep than prey species, and mammals that occupy relatively safe places during sleep (e.g. burrow versus plains dwelling) tend to sleep longer.

This comparative approach to understanding sleep is appealing and will be discussed further below, but a note of caution should be introduced here. Most sleep measures have been obtained from mammals in captivity, where the pressure for obtaining essential resources – food, water, and access to mates – are profoundly altered. Large mammals such as giraffe and elephants in captivity spend approximately 5 hours per day sleeping, but can we expect such patterns of sleep in the wild where these animals migrate great distances over long periods of time? The answer is almost certainly no. Captive versus wild sleep observations in the brown-throated three-toed sloth (*Bradypus variegates*) show that in captivity sloth spend approximately 70% of their time asleep, whilst in the wild estimates of sleep are 40%. (Consider the difference in sleep patterns measured in a 'captive' human in an elderly care home or prison compared to 'freely moving' humans.) Similarly, activity/sleep patterns in mice alter dramatically in the laboratory compared to the wild where they experience food restriction and dramatic changes in light and temperature. The comparative approach to sleep is potentially very valuable, but more field observations, and measurement of NREM–REM in captivity and the wild, are necessary to support further understanding of natural sleep.

Measuring 'natural' sleep in humans is also difficult; not only does it change with age, but it is markedly influenced by modern electric lighting. Access to electricity immediately changes nighttime light exposure and subsequently work and sleep patterns. Important research regarding the pattern, timing, and structure of human sleep 'in the wild' has been pioneered in Brazil. For example, adolescent Brazilians living in an urban environment have significantly later bedtimes (~21:50 hours) on weekdays than rural teenagers without access to electricity (~20:40 hours). The natural pattern and duration of human sleep is essentially unknown; would we really have one consolidated block of 8 hours' sleep in the wild? Urban human sleep patterns are no more natural than those of the laboratory mice.

Why do animals sleep?

The holy grail of sleep biology is to understand why sleep evolved. Gene survival depends upon a species' ability to produce offspring. Those genes that build individuals that in turn out-compete other individuals and produce more offspring will dominate the gene pool of the evolving species. Sleep seems to be associated with huge evolutionary costs; sleeping animals don't eat, drink, or reproduce and are more vulnerable to predation. This high cost implies a critically important adaptive value. So how can sleep serve this purpose? The assumption by many researchers is that there must be a single overarching evolutionary drive for sleep with very ancient roots in our biology. Others reason that there is no single explanation and that different species at different stages of their life cycle will use inactivity/sleep for different reasons, perhaps for energy conservation, or a mechanism to avoid predation, or even for a time to allow recuperative processes to occur. Yet others suggest that sleep is a trait that has no adaptive value but represents a by-product of some other truly adaptive trait yet to be recognized, as, for example, in the cases of the appendix or navel. These arguments notwithstanding, three broad theories have dominated the discussion of why animals sleep, namely a process

Table 2. Sleep across species

Species	Average total sleep time (% of 24 hours)	Average total sleep time (hours/day)
Brown bat	82.9%	19.9
Giant armadillo	75.4%	18.1
North American opossum	75.0%	18.0
Python	75.0%	18.0
Owl monkey	70.8%	17.0
Human (infant)	**66.7%**	**16.0**
Tiger	65.8%	15.8
Tree shrew	65.8%	15.8
Squirrel	62.0%	14.9
Western toad	60.8%	14.6
Ferret	60.4%	14.5
Three-toed sloth	60.0%	14.4
Golden hamster	59.6%	14.3
Platypus	58.3%	14.0
Lion	56.3%	13.5
Gerbil	54.4%	13.1
Rat	52.4%	12.6
Cat	50.6%	12.1
Cheetah	50.6%	12.1
Mouse	50.3%	12.1
Rhesus monkey	49.2%	11.8
Rabbit	47.5%	11.4
Jaguar	45.0%	10.8
Duck	45.0%	10.8
Dog	44.3%	10.6

Bottle-nosed dolphin	43.3%	10.4
Star-nosed mole	42.9%	10.3
Baboon	42.9%	10.3
European hedgehog	42.2%	10.1
Squirrel monkey	41.3%	9.9
Chimpanzee	40.4%	9.7
Guinea pig	39.2%	9.4
Human (adult)	**33.3%**	**8.0**
Pig	32.6%	7.8
Guppy (fish)	29.1%	7.0
Grey seal	25.8%	6.2
Human (elderly)	**22.9%**	**5.5**
Goat	22.1%	5.3
Cow	16.4%	3.9
Asiatic elephant	16.4%	3.9
Sheep	16.0%	3.8
African elephant	13.8%	3.3
Donkey	13.0%	3.1
Horse	12.0%	2.9
Giraffe	7.9%	1.9

that allows (i) cellular restoration; (ii) energy conservation; and (iii) the consolidation of memory and learning.

Cellular restoration–sleep is a process that allows the repair of key cellular components

This theory, in various incarnations, has been around since the time of Aristotle. In support of the hypothesis is the whole notion of sleep rebound and the observation that hard physical exercise causes a moderate increase in NREM sleep. The generalized 'restorative' argument for sleep is sharply contradicted by the fact that during REM sleep, the brain is more active than during wake and many parts of the body remain very active – such as the heart. In addition, individuals who spend the whole day at rest in bed sleep as long (or even longer) than highly active individuals. Cellular restoration has resurfaced in popularity in recent years with the demonstration that a large proportion of genes in the central nervous system change their pattern of expression during sleep, and that much of this change is clearly sleep-driven rather than time of day or circadian-driven. Significantly, many of these sleep-driven changes in gene expression are associated with major metabolic pathways and the replenishment of transmitter vesicles. The attraction of the cellular restoration hypothesis for sleep is that it is universal and can be applied to all animals, including unicellular life. The weakness of the hypothesis is that the gene data are entirely correlative and may not be related to the direct function of sleep, and critically many genes involved in energy metabolism are not affected during sleep. Further, cellular restoration does not explain the complexity and diversity of REM and NREM sleep.

Energy conservation–sleep has evolved to reduce energy demands

Species are not continually active; they have evolved to occupy a temporal niche within the 24-hour day. As a result, diurnal, nocturnal, and crepuscular species may use sleep as an energy-saving device, reducing energy expenditure and foraging during those times when they cannot exploit their environment. In support of this hypothesis, NREM sleep has been shown to be 'hypometabolic' in that it involves a lower metabolic cost than being awake. As metabolic rate increases as mammals get smaller, the prediction would be that sleep should also increase in smaller mammals, which indeed it generally does (Table 2). Modelling approaches also support the idea that even a small energy saving can have an important impact on evolutionary selection, particularly in small mammals in cold climates. In addition, adenosine, which builds up as energy is used while active, has been linked to sleep induction (see Chapter 3).

Calculation of the energy saved by sleep, however, suggests that it is quite modest – the equivalent of a hot dog bun (80 to 130 calories) per night in humans – and it seems unlikely that such a high behavioural price is paid for such small returns. As a result, the intuitive appeal of an energy-saving explanation for sleep is unlikely to be the primary selection pressure for either the evolution or maintenance of sleep in most animal groups. Arguments against highlight the critical point that whilst NREM may be energy-saving, REM sleep results in an increase in brain metabolism. It is also worth stressing that resting conserves almost as much energy as sleep in many species, and aquatic mammals such as whales and dolphins carry on swimming while they sleep, so sleep is clearly not greatly reducing their overall energy expenditure.

While sleep and hibernation have been compared, sleep is fundamentally different from the truly energy-saving states of torpor and hibernation. Hibernation in species like ground squirrels (*Spermophilus* species) involves a dramatic drop in core body temperature to around 0°C and a complete loss of EEG. Interestingly, ectothermic honey bees presented with a temperature gradient between 18°C and 39°C at night selected 23–26°C, suggesting that bees do not choose resting nighttime temperatures that would maximize energy conservation. Arguments against the energy conservation basis for sleep also stress that any saving would be outweighed by the increased vulnerability to predation. Animals are at their most vulnerable when asleep, and notably during REM sleep when they are effectively paralysed. Cows and other large mammals sleep standing during NREM but lie down during REM – increasing their vulnerability further.

Brain efficiency–sleep has evolved for the consolidation of learning and memory

The Earth's rotation generates a profound cycle in both light and temperature, and it seems probable that the very earliest life-forms distributed many of their metabolic functions across the day–night cycle using an endogenous circadian timing mechanism. The evolution of multicellularity, mobility, and complex sensory systems would have been greatly augmented by the ability to learn and memorize experiences. This process is both metabolically expensive and complex, however. To ensure quality control in the establishment of these new brain microcircuits, they would have been laid down during the inactive phase of the rest–activity cycle when metabolic demands were lower and when sensory input was minimal. So sleep evolved as a mechanism for consolidation of specific neuronal networks and is accommodated during that part of the rest–activity cycle when there is sufficient energy and minimal extraneous neural interference and noise – going 'off-line' while the filing is done, as it were.

Evidence from both animal and human studies suggests a strong link between sleep and what has been termed 'sleep-dependent memory processing'. In many animal studies, sleep deprivation after learning tasks has been shown to impair performance in subsequent tests. In humans, procedural learning, declarative learning, and even higher-level 'insight' – the process of mental restructuring in the brain that leads to a sudden gain of understanding or explicit knowledge – have been shown to depend on sleep. The chance of gaining insight is almost three times higher if the individual is allowed to sleep, and some tasks are never learned if sleep is restricted the night after learning. These elegant studies demonstrate that sleep allows the restructuring of new memories (Box 4, Chapter 8).

If sleep allows brains to function at high efficiency by shifting the demanding tasks of neuronal maintenance and memory consolidation to an inactive time, it follows that sessile, slow-moving animals, or animals living in a broadly unchanging uniform environment, would have no requirement for sleep. Interestingly, fish that spend most of their life schooling have been considered not to sleep. One interpretation for this apparent lack of sleep is that the division of labour within the school, with neighbours simply responding in the same manner as each other, decreases an individual's needs for complex information processing. This reduction in sensory processing in an essentially featureless environment negates the need for sleep.

Overall, there is considerable support for the notion that sleep is required for the processing of recently acquired short-term memories (converting some to long-term memory) and the strengthening of long-term memory through changes in brain plasticity and the consolidation of neuronal circuitry. As sleep deprivation impairs cognition, memory, and attention, and sleep has been shown to markedly enhance critical thinking and problem-solving, sleep has been linked to essential neural processing within the higher cortical brain, specifically, consolidating connections made between neurones and the 'pruning back' of connections to leave only the most important ones established when awake. This idea is supported by brain imaging and electrophysiology findings suggesting that learning is associated with the replaying of neuronal circuits during sleep that were initially laid down while awake, and that slow-wave sleep is more intense in those areas of the cortex where the memorization is taking place.

The problems with the consolidation of learning and memory hypothesis are three-fold: (i) the theory relates only to those species with a complex brain; (ii) memory and learning can also occur in the absence of sleep; (iii) if sleep evolved simply to allow the formation and consolidation of memory, then one would predict that those animals with the largest and most complex brains would sleep more. Yet the length of inactivity/sleep does not correlate with a complex nervous system. Some of the longest sleepers include the brown bat, giant armadillo, North American opossum, and python, at 18 hours per day or more (Table 2). So, in summary, whilst sleep may be critical for higher brain function, it cannot be the sole reason why a state of sleep evolved across the animal world.

Sleep versus the rest-activity pattern?

Perhaps the solution to the question of why we sleep requires another approach and should be addressed by asking two separate questions:

(i) What are the selection pressures for the maintenance of a species-specific rest-activity pattern?

(ii) What are the selection pressures for allocating critical 'house-keeping' functions of the body to the different phases of the rest-activity cycle?

As discussed above, the use of the rest or *sleep* phase of the rest-activity cycle for the consolidation of learning and memory would be a classic example of allocating a critical house-keeping function of the brain to the most suitable physiological slot within the 24-hour cycle. Thus, NREM-REM brain EEG provides a description of a specific house-keeping event within the brain, but it does not provide a global definition of sleep across all animal species. This may seem like mere semantics, but it highlights the point that our definition of sleep will greatly influence our understanding of the function of sleep.

The endless discussion regarding the definition of sleep has marginalized the fundamental question of why each species seems to have evolved a specific pattern of rest and activity. The individual selection pressures for 24-hour patterns of rest and activity have, to a large extent, been ignored. In most cases, we don't really know why some species are inactive for 19 hours and others for only 2 hours, but this will certainly arise from a complex set of competing factors such as access to essential resources like food, water, and breeding partners, and of course avoidance of predators, pathogens, and infection. Once an evolutionarily stable rest-activity pattern has evolved for a given species, then essential biological 'house-keeping' processes will be secondarily incorporated into this temporal structure and may well then act to reinforce this framework. As a result, some sleep researchers argue that the EEG merely represents a measure of essential house-keeping functions of the brain that have been allocated to the rest portion of the rest-activity cycle, so that this represents one of many possible surrogate measures of the inactive phase of the rest-activity cycle. Alternatively, other researchers would argue that EEG-defined sleep *is* the inactive portion of the rest-activity cycle. Such alternative views continue to engender fierce debate and will only become resolved when there is an agreed definition of what sleep really represents.

Chapter 5
The seven ages of sleep

We know that our sleep patterns change with age. The hours of blissful uninterrupted sleep that infants enjoy gradually reduces in duration and quality as we age, seemingly reversing into hours of restless interrupted sleep (Table 2). The changes in sleeping patterns throughout life are often difficult to differentiate from changes caused by disorders which are more common in older people, however, and the prevalence of some clinical sleep disorders also changes with age (see Chapter 6), further complicating observation of 'natural' changes in sleep.

Here we have divided the lifespan into seven 'ages' of sleep: sleep during pregnancy, neonatal sleep, sleep in children, sleep in adolescence and young adulthood, sleep during middle age and menopause, sleep in the elderly, and finally sleep–wake disturbance in dementia. These 'ages' are of course artificial – changes in sleep do not occur in discrete episodes but continually throughout life.

Sleep during pregnancy

As any mother will tell you, pregnancy changes sleep: the hormonal changes, physical discomfort and foetal activity, nocturia (excessive urinating at night), leg cramps, and acid reflux all affect the sleep of expectant mums. The risk of sleep disorders also increases, including 'pregnancy-associated sleep disorder' (defined as 'occurrence of either insomnia or excessive sleepiness that develops in the course of pregnancy'), in addition to sleep-disordered breathing and restless legs syndrome.

Most expectant mothers report some sleep disruption, which changes throughout pregnancy. Nighttime sleep and naps increase in the first trimester, with up to an hour more sleep per day, although complaints of sleep disruption and fatigue are also high. This increased sleep duration is likely due to the rapid rise in progesterone secretion which increases sleepiness and body temperature. Sleep disruption then tends to increase as the foetus grows and causes bladder compression and discomfort, and slow-wave and REM sleep may reduce slightly towards the end of pregnancy. The presence of other children or differing experience dealing with a new baby also affect sleep, although feeding method does not show clear associations with new mothers' sleep.

Snoring and shortness of breath increase during pregnancy, possibly due to the effects of progesterone on respiration, although it is unclear whether the incidence of obstructive sleep apnoea (OSA) increases in women who were not at risk before becoming pregnant. It is important to screen for OSA in expectant mothers, however, as left untreated it may increase hypertension and risk of pre-eclampsia and reduce foetal growth. Restless legs syndrome and periodic limb movements also increase during pregnancy with around one-fifth of pregnant women affected, but this can be reduced by supervised treatment with iron and folate. As with many other depressive disorders (Chapter 7), post-partum depression may be associated with greater sleep disruption, although it is not clear whether sleep deprivation during pregnancy increases the risk.

The foetus's rhythms are synchronized to the mother during development. Foetal heart rate is synchronized with the mother's heart rate, sleep, temperature, and melatonin rhythms during the last quarter of gestation. Melatonin, the biochemical signal of darkness, passes through the placenta, and melatonin receptors are present in the neonatal SCN. At least in rodents, the SCN is rhythmic before birth, but the pathways enabling light synchronization of the clock are not yet formed. The establishment of 24-hour circadian rhythms is similarly delayed in humans (see neonatal sleep, below). The foetus still sleeps, however, with distinct episodes of quiet sleep (equivalent to NREM), active sleep (REM), and intermediate sleep as early as 32 weeks.

Neonatal sleep

Sleep becomes a major focus when a child is born – making sure that baby gets a lot while parents try to function with a little. Alongside feeding, sleep dominates every aspect of the new family's life. It is apparent immediately to new parents that babies do not begin life with a stable 24-hour sleep–wake pattern. The circadian clock, which we take for granted as adults, is not yet fully functional in newborns. Newborns initially exhibit 'ultradian' (less than 24-hour) rhythms, with roughly 4-hourly feeds and a seemingly random sleep pattern. As much as 16 hours a day might be spent asleep in the first few weeks of life. Over the first few months, sleep still dominates but gradually becomes more consolidated, with fewer but longer sleep bouts. The homeostatic control of sleep is apparent relatively early on and, while it is difficult for parents to notice, baby's circadian system also starts to become functional around this time. The clock begins to generate non-24-hour sleep–wake rhythms but cannot yet be synchronized to the 24-hour light–dark cycle (Figure 9). After 2–6 months, however, a distinct 24-hour cycle emerges, with a major nighttime sleep episode and shorter naps in the daytime, which stabilizes at 6–12 months of age (Figure 9). Melatonin is passed in breast milk, and if night-milk is given at night (rather than pumped in the day and

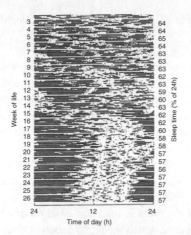

9. The sleep–wake cycle takes several months to become stably synchronized. At the start of life, an ultradian (<24 hour) or arrhythmic pattern in sleep (black lines) and feeding (dots) is apparent, before gradually developing a non-24-hour rhythm, and finally synchronizes to the 24-hour day some time in the first 3–6 months

given at night), this might provide a synchronizing time cue in early life.

Childhood sleep has a different structure to adult sleep and changes substantially throughout development. The NREM-REM sleep cycle lasts only 60 minutes in babies, and there is much more REM sleep than in adults. At 2 weeks of age, half of the sleep episode consists of REM sleep, reducing to about one-third by 6 months of age. It has been suggested that increased REM sleep is necessary for consolidating the vast amounts of new information that needs to be learned and memorized as babies begin to take in the world around them. Both REM and NREM sleep play a key role in brain maturation, and therefore getting adequate sleep is vitally important in neonatal cognitive development.

Stable 24-hour rhythms are virtually impossible to achieve in the first few weeks of life, given the necessity of regular feeds and the lack of a strong circadian control of sleep. Even at this early stage, however, the sleep environment should still be maintained in a way to encourage sleep and eventually to help synchronize the biological clock. The sleeping environment should be as dark as possible – use black-out curtains or even aluminium foil to block out light – and night-lights should be avoided. If night-lights must be used, use the dimmest red light possible and limit the time that it is on. Ensure the room is quiet and avoid playing tunes to soothe children to sleep, or switch them off as soon as sleep begins. As the baby gets older, develop a stable schedule with a strong 24-hour pattern of light days and dark nights.

More specific advice on what to do to help babies get to sleep and stay asleep is a matter of great debate, fuelled by dozens of self-help books, and is beyond the scope of this chapter. One common approach is 'self-soothing' for babies aged 4–6 months whereby parents are encouraged not to immediately soothe their baby when they wake and cry, allowing them to soothe themselves for increasing durations, starting with short bursts of several minutes and increasing the time gradually over days and weeks. Opponents of this method suggest that it is stressful for the infant and affects parental trust, and may desensitize parents to babies' cries; they prefer to encourage 'parental soothing' whereby parents rock, nurse, or sing their child back to sleep. The best general advice is to do what works, and several methods may need to be tried before an effective one is found.

While babies' sleep is vitally important for their health and development, parental sleep is also of concern for everybody's health and safety. New parents experience substantial sleep deprivation and need to consider the potential risk that this poses for drowsy driving and accidents at work and home (Chapter 8), and in particular the inadvisable practice of driving children around to get them to sleep. The effects of sleep deprivation on psychological health also place new parents and their relationship under additional stress, with sometimes dangerous consequences – many parents will describe being 'pushed to the edge' by lack of sleep and infants' continuous crying. The dangers of sleep deprivation are poorly recognized by both unsympathetic non-parents and memory-challenged 'former' parents, and, while sleep disruption cannot be avoided, increased awareness and prioritization of parental sleep should be a focus for health professionals and support networks when new children arrive. Strategies might include regularly going to bed early, taking naps when baby naps (leave the ironing!), and asking family and friends to help for a few hours while you sleep. If a long trip is coming up, ensure that the driver gets several full nights of sleep by sleeping in a separate room. Take every opportunity to sleep, and to sleep in the right environment. These strategies will not solve the problem completely, but moving sleep higher in the priority list will help.

Sleep in children

How much sleep do children need? The answer is as much as possible. Sleep should have the highest priority and be actively sought and protected by parents. Sleep is vitally important for the health and development of children, and we are yet to understand the long-term, and possibly life-time, consequences of insufficient sleep in early life.

Total sleep duration reduces through childhood, with a median sleep duration of 8–9 hours by late adolescence, falling from about 16 hours in the first few months of life (although ranging from 9 to 19 hours). The NREM–REM cycle gradually extends from 60 minutes in newborns, to 75 minutes at 2 years, and reaches the 90-minute sleep cycle seen in adults by around 6 years of age. The proportion of sleep spent in slow-wave and REM sleep reduces with age, mirrored by an increase in stage 2 sleep. External factors also affect sleep in children, particularly early school start times, which curtail sleep opportunity (Chapter 8). These problems appear to be getting worse: for example, 3-year-olds in the US lost 25 minutes of sleep per night, or nearly 3 hours a week, between the 1970s and 1990s. Given that parents have more control over bedtime than wake-time, these changes are likely induced by – but then can also be corrected by – failure to prioritize sleep.

Napping is often a concern to parents of young children in deciding how many, how long, and at what age to reduce them. Sleeping in the day would theoretically reduce sleep likelihood at night, if there were no residual tiredness, but this is unlikely. Most children (and adults) are not getting enough sleep, and therefore reducing napping may deprive children of much-needed recovery if they are not getting their entire sleep need fulfilled at night. Napping should be age-appropriate and a reduction in daytime naps should be accompanied by a gradual increase in sleep opportunity at night so that the child has the chance to make up for the lost sleep in the day. The extended sleep opportunity should be scheduled for several weeks until the parent understands what the child's maximum sleep need is.

As with babies, there are myriad books and self-help websites to advise parents on their children's sleep. Such advice is beyond the scope of this book, but there are a number of important considerations which are sometimes overlooked. Difficulty falling asleep and bedtime resistance, more formally termed 'behavioural insomnia of childhood', is difficult for children and carers and requires good sleep hygiene practices. Bedtime rituals not only help condition the child to go to sleep, they also help to synchronize the circadian clock and maintain a more regular sleep–wake pattern. Particularly important are the lighting conditions before and during sleep. Bright light immediately before bedtime will alert the brain and may shift the clock to a later time, making it more difficult to go to sleep. The pre-bedtime ritual should occur in as dim a light as possible and removed when asleep. Use of dim, incandescent or redder light sources are preferable, and the new bright 'bluer' LED-type of light should be avoided in the bedroom. Note that going to bed too early may impinge on the 'wake maintenance zone' (Chapter 2) and exacerbate difficulties with sleep onset, but this can be monitored and avoided with experience. Children should also avoid caffeine, which is a powerful stimulant and can significantly impair sleep (Chapter 8).

Sleep deprivation can also cause over-activation, and while there is as yet limited causal evidence linking sleep disruption to behavioural problems or attention and hyperactivity disorders in children, chronic sleep deficiency is likely to exacerbate problem behaviours. As every parent knows, over-tired children act up and have temper tantrums, and are moody, irritable, and sometimes aggressive, and it is not difficult to imagine that repeated failure to obtain sufficient sleep, especially if coupled with caffeine intake, may exacerbate poor behaviour.

There is another increasingly important challenge to sleep in childhood. Childhood obesity is rising dramatically in industrialized nations and brings with it an increased risk of obstructive sleep apnoea (OSA) which, while not specific to children, may have a greater potential health impact so early in life. As described in Chapter 6, OSA is a serious disorder in which the airway collapses during sleep, temporarily suffocating the individual, which causes them to wake in order to breathe. These episodes, or 'apnoeas', can occur dozens of times an hour in serious cases and prevent the sufferer from obtaining any deep restorative sleep. OSA risk increases with weight gain, and therefore an epidemic of childhood obesity will inevitably lead to an epidemic of childhood OSA. Children also have the additional complication of enlarged tonsils which also increases OSA risk. Children with OSA cannot obtain sufficient sleep, and as a result have more daytime sleepiness, more aggression and oppositional behaviour, learning and memory difficulties, and increased rates of anxiety, depression, and hyperactivity. There is also evidence of increased cardiometabolic disorders, as seen in adults (Chapter 6).

Sleep in adolescence and young adulthood

As parents are well aware, sleep patterns change dramatically during adolescence. Sleep becomes delayed, with bedtimes occurring late into the night and wake times sometimes pushing into the afternoon. These problems occur because of changes in the control of sleep that delays teenagers' sleep propensity to a later time. These biological changes often put teenagers at odds with societal and parental expectations and lead to misplaced accusations of laziness or deliberate misbehaviour.

Adolescents experience a delay in their sleep and circadian rhythms, with a 2–3 hour change in the timing of their clocks over their teenage years, correlating closely with pubertal development. Children, particularly males, gradually become more 'evening type' throughout their teenage years until their early 20s, after which they start to advance, males slightly lagging the females. The prevalence of delayed sleep phase disorder, a circadian rhythm sleep disorder characterized by extremely delayed sleep–wake timing (Chapter 6), is also highest during adolescence, at about 15%.

This shift is not due to a lengthening of the body clock period but due to a change in the timing between circadian and homeostatic control of sleep. In addition to phase delaying, older teenagers tend to have reduced slow-wave sleep and have a slower rate of sleep pressure build-up during the day, and therefore take longer to build up the critical homeostatic level of sleepiness required to induce sleep. Parents will recognize that younger children reach their critical threshold for falling sleep much earlier.

So what are the consequences of this sleep shift? Young adults need lots of sleep – at least 8.5 hours a night when given unlimited opportunity to sleep, and more for teenagers. Given that not all time in bed is spent asleep, teenagers going to sleep at midnight, 1 a.m., or later do not have the opportunity to get 8.5 hours sleep before they have to get up for school, resulting in a dramatic curtailing of their sleep 5 days a week. When they try and sleep according to their natural cycle at weekends, they are harangued for being lazy and made to get up, or are 'missing the best part of the day'. Despite the potential seriousness of these problems, older (phase-advanced) adults often dismiss such social 'jetlag' and this conflict between adolescents' biology and societal expectations is having significant consequences on the health, development, and safety of adolescents and young adults (Chapters 7 and 8).

How might these conflicts be minimized? Parents must recognize that later sleep is biologically based; while computer games and TVs may reinforce late sleep times, they are not the underlying cause. Understanding the severity of the problem is also key; teenagers are essentially living in another time zone, so having teenagers get up for school at 7 a.m. is like asking adults to wake at 4 a.m., and so it is not surprising that teenagers are unresponsive and irritated. Modest delays in school start times can have a major effect on academic performance and behaviour (Chapter 8). Protecting time for sleep, particularly at weekends, is important, as is monitoring of late-evening extracurricular activities, caffeine use, and other factors that reduce sleep. While it is difficult for the delay to be entirely corrected, gradually advancing bedtimes, and reducing activities and light exposure prior to bed may help shift bedtimes earlier and increase sleep opportunities. As with younger children, sleep should be prioritized and taken at every opportunity. Lead by example: prioritize the entire family's sleep, including your own, as developing good attitudes towards sleep in early adulthood will hopefully lead to better sleep habits throughout life.

Middle age and menopause

Our sleep changes continually throughout adulthood. We become more morning-type as the timing of the circadian pacemaker gradually advances, and our sleep duration reduces, including the proportion of slow-wave and REM sleep. There is a reduction in the robustness of the homeostatic regulation of sleep, contributing to greater difficulties recovering from sleep deprivation or unusual work shifts. Gender differences in sleep and sleep perception also tend to become more apparent in middle age, with women generally having more complaints about sleep than men, despite getting more sleep, including more deep sleep, when measured objectively (Figure 1). Social factors also encroach on our sleep opportunities as we try to balance family life with career aspirations, squeezing out sleep, and the risk of clinical sleep disorders increases as we age, particularly due to weight gain (obstructive sleep apnoea) or the stresses of life (insomnia) (Chapter 6).

Menopause has major effects on sleep, inducing symptoms that affect sleep including night sweats and mood disorders, in addition to long sleep latencies and reduced slow-wave sleep. Post-menopausal women have nearly double the rate of insomnia complaints as pre-menopausal women, although when sleep is measured objectively, these differences are reversed, suggesting that hormonal status may also affect sleep-state misperception. OSA risk is three times higher after the menopause, most likely due to hormone-related redistribution of fat, and this appears to be reduced in women taking hormone replacement therapy (HRT).

Sleep in the elderly

Many people experience poorer sleep as they get older and accept it as an inevitable result of ageing. Consequently, older people are thought to need less sleep or to be incapable of getting good sleep.

In healthy ageing, however, sleep need not necessarily be substantially impaired, although some changes do occur. The prevalence of many medical and psychiatric conditions that affect sleep increases with age, as does medication use. The risk of some sleep disorders is also age-related (Chapter 6).

As we age, consolidation of both sleep and wakefulness reduces, with more broken sleep and increased likelihood of daytime naps. It takes older people a little longer to fall asleep, and there is a reduction in sleep 'depth' with less slow-wave and REM sleep and an increase in stage 1 and 2 sleep. Awakenings are also more frequent, leading to a reduction in sleep time and sleep efficiency. Sleep timing generally continues to advance, and older people rate themselves as more morning-type. As with teenagers, this shift is not due to a change in the natural period of the circadian pacemaker – the clock remains stable in healthy ageing – but due to changes in how the circadian and homeostatic processes controlling sleep interact. The circadian 'window' for sleep narrows with old age, limiting the duration of time that prolonged, consolidated sleep can be achieved. This results in older people waking at an earlier phase of their circadian cycle than younger adults. This narrowing of the sleep opportunity is reflected in the maximum sleep that older adults can obtain; when extended sleep opportunities are provided, older people (≥ 60 years) sleep about 7.5 hours maximally, about an hour less than young people under similar circumstances. It is not clear whether this represents sleep 'need' in terms of what is biologically required to maintain optimal function, but does represent at least the biological capacity to sleep. Failure to achieve these totals on a daily basis – defined as chronic sleep deficiency – is likely to result in a progressive decline in alertness and performance over time. Interestingly, however, healthy older people appear to be less affected by acute sleep deprivation than younger subjects, who generally find it more difficult to stay awake and perform well for 24 hours or more, and this may explain the high rate of drowsy-driving car crashes among young people (Chapter 8).

It is often stated that older people have more sleep problems because they produce less of the nighttime hormone melatonin (Chapter 2). On average, older people have lower melatonin levels than younger individuals due to the reduced capacity of the pineal gland to produce melatonin, and/or an overall reduction in the amplitude of circadian rhythms. Healthy older subjects have melatonin levels and rhythms as robust as younger subjects, however, suggesting that the melatonin decline may be a consequence of some pathology. Melatonin 'replacement therapy' – giving synthetic melatonin as a sleeping aid to older people – is not successful at improving sleep, suggesting that low levels of melatonin are not in themselves the cause of sleep problems. Strengthening circadian rhythmicity by exposing oneself to a robust light–dark cycle, however, does have potential for improving sleep and behaviour in older people, as discussed in the section on dementia below.

There are other factors associated with ageing that also potentially affect sleep. As we age, the lens in the eye gradually yellows due to pigment deposition, and this changes the transmission of light through the lens and reduces the amount of short-wavelength, or blue, light that gets through. Blue light is the most effective wavelength for resetting the circadian clock (Chapter 2), and therefore reductions in blue light exposure might increase the risk of developing circadian rhythm sleep disorders and explain why older people are more phase-advanced. Similar considerations apply to cataracts, which block light across the entire spectrum, although there is debate about the best type of replacement lens to use. Intraocular lenses are available that mimic either the yellower ageing lens or a young lens that lets the blue light through. While the latter may be expected to help circadian sleep problems, some researchers argue that failure to block blue light increases the risk of eye damage, particularly the risk of age-related macular degeneration (ARMD), a common eye disorder in older people, especially in those who have worked outside. A number of studies are currently addressing this question, so the jury is still out on the best approach.

Temperature regulation is a key factor in falling and staying asleep, and poor temperature regulation is associated with sleep complaints. Poor circulation is one potential cause and may be associated with sleep complaints in older people. As we go to sleep, core body temperature falls more quickly than the natural circadian decline, and is accompanied by increased heat loss at our extremities (hands and feet). People with poor circulation and cold hands and feet cannot lose as much heat and take longer to get to sleep. Warming the hands and feet, which causes vasodilation and increases body heat loss, increases sleepiness and increases the likelihood of falling asleep. So Grandma was right – bed socks and a night-cap are a good idea, as they will increase overall heat loss and help you get to sleep.

Dementia

Although dementia is not an inevitable consequence of ageing, it is prevalent in older people, with up to 50% of those aged 85 years or older affected. Approximately two-thirds of cases are due to Alzheimer's disease, the leading cause of dementia.

To some extent, ageing and dementia share symptoms of disrupted sleep–wake and rest–activity cycles which in themselves may exacerbate cognitive decline. The number of cells in the circadian pacemaker declines modestly with ageing but reduces significantly in Alzheimer's disease and is accompanied by a dramatic loss of rhythmic amplitude by clock cells. The reduced strength of the rhythmic signal from these cells may underlie the weakening of daily rhythms observed in very old people and dementia patients. Disordered rest–activity patterns are the main reason for institutionalizing a dementia patient, due to both the physical risk of wandering about at night and chronic sleep disruption for the carer. Early home-based treatment of the rest–activity disturbance in those with mild to moderate dementia may therefore delay when a patient needs to go into care.

A promising approach to deal with dementia-related rest–activity disorder is to address the lack of a robust light–dark cycle that is often experienced by patients and the elderly, particularly those living in care homes. In a large prospective Dutch study, dementia patients in care homes where the indoor lighting was simply increased to about 1,000 lux from 10 a.m. to 6 p.m. (compared to standard lighting at about 300 lux) exhibited a significant slowing in the rate of cognitive decline, improved day-to-day functioning, less depression, and better sleep. These improvements were equivalent to those obtained with prescription medication therapy. While the exact mechanism of action is unknown, light has acute alerting properties in addition to its circadian resetting effects, and therefore better daytime lighting may improve arousal and cognitive function. A more robust light–dark cycle will also stabilize sleep–wake patterns and improve sleep, which in itself may help slow the decline in cognitive function. Light also has mood-elevating and clinical antidepressant effects in some conditions, such as seasonal affective disorder, which may account for the lower depression ratings.

This approach is not a panacea for all symptoms of dementia, but it is a simple, non-invasive, and inexpensive approach to encourage good sleep–wake patterns and better sleep, and potentially reduce the rate of cognitive decline and depression. This approach is not limited to those with dementia; reinforcing daily light–dark patterns in all elderly people, especially those who do not get outside daily, is likely to be of benefit, as is reinforcing good light–dark cycles in hospitals and other care facilities, schools and colleges, and our own homes. From newborns to old age, maximizing dark nights and light days is key for good sleep and circadian rhythm regulation.

Chapter 6
When sleep suffers

When we sleep well, we take it for granted. Unfortunately, about one-third of us will suffer from at least one of around 75 clinical sleep disorders at some time during our lives. Many will have sleep problems without receiving a formal diagnosis. Such sleep disorders may be temporary, perhaps as a result of a traumatic experience such as bereavement or divorce, or can become a chronic, lifelong problem. Some are brought on by people's own behaviour, for example by working at night or gaining too much weight, or can be associated with other factors such as pain, disease, or medication use. Regardless of the cause, sleep disorders dramatically affect quality of life and, long term, are detrimental to health and wellbeing. Most people don't realize the benefits that sleep brings until they can't sleep well any more.

There are eight types of sleep disorders according to the *International Classification of Sleep Disorders* (ICSD-2):
I. insomnia; II. sleep-related breathing disorders; III. hypersomnia of central origin; IV. circadian rhythm sleep disorders;
V. parasomnias; VI. sleep-related movement disorders; VII. isolated symptoms and normal variants; VIII. other sleep disorders. A full review of all sleep disorders is not possible here, but the Further reading section lists more detailed books. We will discuss the most common disorders and those that have the greatest impact on health and society.

Insomnia

Insomnia is not a specific disease but a broad symptom describing inability to sleep and it is the most common sleep complaint. It encompasses different sleep problems; some patients find it difficult to fall asleep (sleep-onset insomnia), some can fall asleep easily but cannot stay asleep (sleep-maintenance insomnia), and some wake up too early. Transient insomnia can start and end quite quickly in relation to a life event, whereas some individuals will have a lifelong battle with insomnia, never feeling able to get enough sleep. Insomnia is associated with many psychiatric conditions (see Chapter 7) and can be associated with other problems such as pain, disorders such as rheumatoid arthritis and Parkinson's disease, heartburn, or alcohol and drug abuse. Some insomniacs have a disconnect between their perceived amount of sleep or sleep need and how much they actually get, termed 'sleep state misperception' or 'paradoxical insomnia', and insomnia patients sometimes sleep more than they think. Patients often do not feel restored in the morning and may report sleepiness, fatigue, or malaise, problems with attention, concentration and performance, poor mood, low energy or irritability, drowsy-related accidents at work or while driving, or a general anxiety about sleep. For a clinical diagnosis, these symptoms must usually persist for at least a month.

Up to 40% of adults may suffer from insomnia at some time in their lives, with as many as 15% suffering chronically. Women report more insomnia than men, although women actually tend to sleep better when measured in studies. Insomnia complaints increase with age, with as many as half of over-65s reporting problems. Sleep is also often disturbed in older people by having to get up to go to the bathroom at least once a night, a situation termed 'nocturia', which affects more than one-third of older people (and some younger adults), and, when chronic, is associated with poor health outcomes and increased mortality.

There are multiple causes of insomnia, but patients generally fall into three categories. Some individuals appear to have an inherent predisposition for insomnia and may exhibit hyperarousal or a low homeostatic drive for sleep, making it difficult to fall asleep or maintain sleep. There may also be precipitating factors that increase the incidence of insomnia, including life events, diseases, nocturia, medications, and drugs or alcohol. Finally, individuals may perpetuate behaviours that lead to insomnia, such as use of televisions and computers in the bedroom; exercising, eating, or seeing bright light late in the evening; caffeine overuse; napping in the day; or worrying about sleep, which may in turn make sleep more difficult. The latter problem can become a conditioned response – 'learned' insomnia – whereby patients get into a vicious cycle in which they have acute insomnia due to a life event or start worrying about whether they can sleep, which leads to difficulties with falling asleep, which leads to further worry and behaviours which delay sleep or make it more difficult, which leads to more worries about sleep, and so on. Breaking this cycle is an important component of insomnia therapy and includes removing the perpetuating factors and improving sleep hygiene.

Untreated insomnia is associated with health problems, although the mechanisms are not known; some diseases may lead to insomnia symptoms, or insomnia may develop as the primary disorder and then increase the risk of subsequently developing other diseases. Insomnia or insufficient sleep is associated with increased risk of heart disease, stroke, and depression. Insomnia is also a common symptom in psychiatric disorders (Chapter 7). Treatment of sleep problems, while not addressing the primary cause of the psychiatric disorder, may improve functioning in patients by improving daytime sleepiness and mood, or provide a better daily structure.

Treatment options vary depending on the underlying cause of the insomnia. Addressing an initial cause of insomnia, such as better pain management or recovery from bereavement, can relieve the symptoms. In primary insomnia, however, therapies that address the insomnia itself are required, and the most common non-pharmaceutical approaches include stimulus control, sleep restriction, and relaxation therapy, and some or all of these may be combined with cognitive behavioural therapy (CBT). These approaches aim to restructure sleeping habits and dismantle conditioned behaviours contributing to the insomnia. Under supervision over several weeks, patients address any anxiety contributing to the insomnia and develop better sleep habits by keeping a more consistent sleep–wake schedule, performing relaxation techniques before bed, removing stimulants such as television, computers, telephones, personal organizers, and light from the bedroom, and rescheduling caffeine use and exercise earlier in the day. When they cannot sleep, patients are discouraged from lying awake for hours in bed but are advised to get up and do some low-level activity in dim light elsewhere before repeating the procedure for going to bed. Sleep-restriction techniques are also used, whereby patients are scheduled to be in bed initially for a restricted amount of time (for example, for 6 hours) to maintain a high sleep efficiency and reduce the amount of time lying awake, which is then gradually expanded until longer durations of high-efficiency sleep are achieved. These techniques are designed to break bad habits and replace them with good sleep hygiene (Table 3). CBT has a high degree of long-term success if patients are compliant.

Hypnotic medication, or 'sleeping pills', are commonly used in the treatment of insomnia, with more than 10 million prescriptions for hypnotics written annually in England alone. A range of medications have sleep-inducing effects, and older approaches to insomnia treatment included non-approved use of tranquillizers, sedating antidepressants, and antipsychotic medication in non-depressed patients. Today, most modern hypnotics approved for treating insomnia are short-acting benzodiazepines (such as Temazepam, Triazolam, Estazolam) and the so-called 'Z-drugs', which act in a benzodiazepine-like manner but are chemically different (Zaleplon, Zolpidem, Zopiclone, Eszopiclone). These drugs have varying half-lives (time taken for the concentration in the body to decrease by

Table 3. 'Sleep hygiene' tips for healthy people

DON'T	DO
Have a television in the bedroom or watch television in bed	Try to go to bed and get up at the same time each day
Use the computer in the bedroom or sleep with electronic devices by the bed	Restrict the use of the bedroom to sleep and sex
Argue or do vigorous exercise just before bed	Get regular exercise each day, preferably in the morning/afternoon
Have caffeine in the late afternoon or evening	Get regular exposure to outdoor light
Use alcohol or other aids to help you sleep	Keep the temperature in the bedroom cool
Go to bed too hungry or too full	Keep the bedroom quiet when sleeping and use ear plugs
Take another person's sleeping pills	Keep the bedroom completely dark using black-out curtains or use an eye-mask
Take over-the-counter medications to aid sleep (e.g. antihistamines)	Keep your feet and hands warm and use bedsocks
Take daytime naps longer than 20 mins	Take short daytime naps
Use a nightlight, but if you need one, use as dim a red-orange light as possible	Have the lights as dim as possible in the hour or two before bed
Become anxious about not sleeping	Do something relaxing before you go to bed such as relaxation exercises, meditation, have a warm bath or warm non-caffeinated drink
Be pressured by others regarding your sleep needs and times	Listen to your body about the amount of sleep you need

half; a measure of duration of effect), with the most common ranging from 1 to 11 hours, and therefore drug choice needs to be balanced between obtaining sufficiently long sleep versus potential adverse effects on daytime functioning, particularly the risk of morning falls in the elderly and impaired driving ability. Amnesia after waking in the night is also a potential risk with some of the medications which may make them inappropriate under certain circumstances.

Current guidelines recommend use for several weeks only, although people are often prescribed them for much longer and risk developing drug dependency. Patients sometimes feel the need to increase their dose to get the same effect (often without permission) and can then experience withdrawal symptoms and rebound insomnia when stopping the medication. More recently, melatonin and melatonin receptor agonists have been approved for insomnia treatment, and these do not have the same risk of dependence but can have limited effectiveness.

About 40% of patients with insomnia also self-medicate with alcohol, over-the-counter sleep aids and medications, or untested herbal remedies. Alcohol is often used to help people to fall asleep, although alcohol's effectiveness in facilitating sleep quickly reduces over time and consumption increases sleep disturbance due to nocturia. Some antihistamines induce sleepiness by blocking the histaminergic alerting effects in the brain (Chapter 3).

Some medications and substances may also contribute to insomnia, including central nervous system stimulants, some antihypertensive and respiratory medications, decongestants, hormone replacement therapy, chemotherapy drugs, diet pills, nicotine, and caffeine (Chapter 3).

Sleep-related breathing disorders

Sleep-related breathing disorders account for a high proportion of sleep complaints. The most common is obstructive sleep apnoea

(OSA) syndrome which is characterized by a repeated partial or complete closing of the airway (an apnoea) when patients lie down to sleep, cutting off the air supply and causing them to start to suffocate and then to wake up. Apnoeas are often followed by a noisy gasp, which the bed partner often hears. This goes beyond simply snoring, although heavy snorers are at risk of OSA. An apnoea is defined as a reduction of air flow by at least 90% for at least 10 seconds (30% for a hypopnoea) accompanied by a fall of blood oxygen levels by 3–4%. Having 15 or more of these events an hour (an Apnoea-Hypopnoea Index, AHI, of 15 or higher) warrants a formal diagnosis of OSA, but having at least 5 events per hour is considered 'mild' OSA and may still have health consequences. Thirty events an hour or more is categorized as 'severe', and in very serious cases, patients stop breathing as often as 100 times an hour. Such regular sleep disruption prevents patients getting into the deep slow-wave sleep that restores alertness and they are therefore often very tired and exhibit cognitive problems. Drowsy-driving crashes are a particular risk in this patient group, with up to a 7-fold risk of accidents if they remain untreated. The repeated shock of being woken abruptly every few minutes also makes heart rate more variable, raising blood pressure and increasing the risk of stroke and heart attack; untreated OSA patients have a 2–3-fold increase in the risk of dying from a heart attack or stroke. They also have an increased risk of insulin resistance and diabetes.

OSA is highly prevalent in middle-aged, overweight patients, particularly men, although post-menopausal women are also at high risk. Obesity (usually defined by body mass index (BMI), the ratio of weight to height, kg/m^2, of 30 or higher) and large neck size are strong indicators of OSA risk, as the increased fat around the neck 'crushes' the airway when lying down to sleep. At higher BMIs, OSA is virtually guaranteed. Given the high risk of drowsy-driving crashes in untreated OSA patients, it has been proposed that all commercial drivers with high BMIs be required to complete OSA screening and treatment before being issued a driving licence. In the interests of public safety, one could consider applying this requirement to all drivers, not just commercial truck drivers, and to pilots, ships' captains, train drivers, and to other safety-related professions involving contact with the public (e.g. police, firefighters, doctors, nurses). Targeted OSA screening programmes would benefit both individual health and public safety.

OSA not only occurs in obese patients, however. Lean people can also have OSA due to anatomical changes that occlude the airway, including a short airway that easily collapses under pressure, a large tongue or oversized tonsils that partially block the airway, or an unusual jaw shape.

A range of treatments are available, the most common being continuous positive airway pressure (CPAP), during which the patient wears a small mask over their nose or mouth that pushes air down the airway during sleep to ensure that it stays open. Although it may take a few days to get used to wearing the mask, CPAP therapy can be very successful and is non-invasive and relatively simple. Weight loss is also often recommended as an initial approach to treat OSA. Other approaches may be more appropriate, depending on the cause: dental devices can be worn to help stop the tongue blocking the airway or reposition the jaw slightly, and a small number of patients may require surgery to remove the tonsils or reshape the jaw. Patients successfully treated for OSA often notice changes in daytime alertness and cognition, and come to realize how sleepy and run-down they felt before.

Central sleep apnoea syndromes are a related but less common group of disorders in which breathing becomes disordered during sleep. In contrast to OSA, the airway remains open during central apnoeas but the person makes an abnormal, or even no, effort to breathe. This can be caused by a variety of problems including changes in the nervous system regulation of breathing during sleep, lung disease, or cardiovascular disease, for example in congestive heart failure or after a stroke. These disorders are associated with reduced responses to events that should automatically trigger greater breathing effort, such as an apnoea or raised levels of carbon dioxide in the blood, which results in disrupted sleep. Similar problems are seen in people travelling to high altitude.

Hypersomnia of central origin

Disorders in this category describe symptoms of excessive daytime sleepiness (hypersomnia) that are not due to sleep apnoea, circadian disorders, or other sleep problems but are due to an intrinsic, 'central' disorder in the brain. Three types of disorder have been described and the best understood of these is narcolepsy – literally 'sleep attacks' – which is characterized by being irresistibly overcome by sleep (even when active), regular napping, and excessive daytime sleepiness. Nighttime sleep is also fragmented, with less consolidated sleep, and patients may experience REM paralysis or intrusion of an REM-like state into wakefulness. Narcolepsy subtypes are described, specifically narcolepsy with or without cataplexy, and narcolepsy due to a medical condition (such as head trauma, Parkinson's disease, or multiple sclerosis). Cataplexy is a sudden loss of muscle tone that can cause patients to literally crumple in a heap, temporarily paralysed, while remaining awake for up to several minutes, and is often triggered by intense emotional responses such as laughter, surprise, or occasionally anger. Cataplexy can be a frightening condition, although some patients have less severe, localized symptoms, such as a temporarily slackened jaw or weakness at the knees.

Narcolepsy is rare, affecting less than 0.2% of the population, but can be a disabling disorder. Important advances have been made recently in understanding the basis of narcolepsy. As reviewed in Chapter 3, orexin/hypocretin is a key component of the sleep–wake regulatory system. Activation of orexin neurones drives wakefulness, and low levels of orexin at night drive sleep. Orexin has been described as the 'finger' on a flip-flop switch, controlling the rate of transition between sleep and wakeful states and helping to maintain episodes of consolidated wakefulness or sleep.

Narcoleptic patients have very low orexin levels and few orexin-producing cells, and therefore lose this important control mechanism for maintaining a normal sleep–wake pattern. While there is not yet a cure, some of the symptoms can be treated, for example by using stimulants to counter excessive sleepiness.

The other hypersomnias, idiopathic hypersomnia (daytime sleepiness without known cause) and recurrent hypersomnia (recurring bouts of daytime sleepiness and other cognitive dysfunction), are rare and not well understood. Recurrent hypersomnia occurs in Kleine-Levine syndrome along with recurrent behavioural disorders including binge-eating and hypersexuality as well as cognitive impairment, irritability, and aggression. Hypersomnia associated with the menstrual cycle also falls into this category. In idiopathic hypersomnia, patients have excessive daytime sleepiness and unrefreshing naps, and often suffer severe sleep inertia upon waking. Some patients also have very long nighttime sleep episodes. There may be autoimmune or genetic bases to these disorders, but treatments are currently limited to addressing the daytime sleepiness symptoms.

Circadian rhythm sleep disorders

Circadian rhythm sleep disorders (CRSD) are caused by sleep being attempted or occurring at an abnormal time in the circadian cycle (Figure 10). There is only a narrow window of time within the daily cycle when sleep can easily be initiated and maintained; attempting to sleep outside of this window results in difficulty falling or staying asleep. Circadian rhythm sleep disorders can be self-induced, environmentally induced, or due to an intrinsic disorder in the circadian organization of sleep. They can be particularly prevalent in certain groups, such as delayed sleep phase disorder in adolescents, advanced sleep phase disorder in elderly people, non-24-hour sleep–wake disorder in totally blind people, and irregular sleep–wake disorder in dementia patients (Chapter 5).

Causes of insomnia (a) and sleepiness (b) in night-shift workers

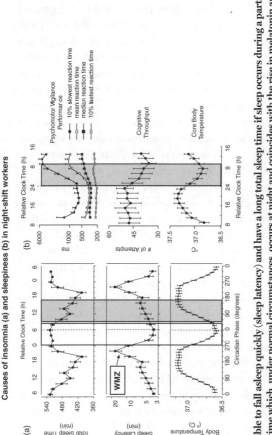

10. (a) It is only possible to fall asleep quickly (sleep latency) and have a long total sleep time if sleep occurs during a particular window of circadian time which, under normal circumstances, occurs at night and coincides with the rise in melatonin and the fall in core body temperature. Trying to sleep too early means that the sleep attempt coincides with the wake maintenance zone (WMZ) which makes it harder to fall asleep. When sleeps occurs at completely the wrong circadian time, for example when a shift-worker sleeps in the middle of the day (grey panel), sleep latency is long and sleep duration is reduced. (b) Similarly, performance also demonstrates a circadian rhythm, and performance levels are high in the day and low at night. Nightshift-workers stay awake during the night when performance is poor (grey panel), increasing the risk of sleepiness-related accidents

Treatment of CRSDs requires changing the timing of sleep so that it occurs at the correct circadian phase, or resetting and maintaining the circadian pacemaker in alignment with the desired time for sleep. The most powerful synchronizing agents are the light–dark cycle and melatonin treatment, although formal clinical guidelines for their therapeutic use are limited. Light and melatonin are considered 'chronobiotics' – treatments that shift the clock and have a different effect depending on the time of day of administration. The direction and magnitude of their effects are described by phase response curves (PRC) – for example, light administration in the late evening shifts the circadian pacemaker to a later time (delay), whereas early morning exposure shifts the clock earlier (advance). Melatonin treatment has a different PRC – melatonin administration in the evening advances the clock whereas morning melatonin causes delays. These properties can be used to time light–dark or melatonin treatment to shift the clock in the desired direction; for advanced sleep phase disorder, evening light and morning melatonin will shift the clock later, whereas morning light and evening melatonin would advance the clock in treating delayed sleep phase disorder (Figure 11). Both natural daylight and light 'boxes' can be used in treating CRSDs, and minimizing light exposure at the wrong time is also important to avoid undoing the desired effects (Chapter 9). Melatonin is available on prescription in most countries (and over the counter in the USA), but most doctors are not trained in how to time it. Many patients therefore do not get the potential benefits of melatonin because it is often timed incorrectly; clearer clinical guidelines are needed. Melatonin and melatonin-like drugs (called 'agonists') also have a mild 'soporific', or sleep-facilitating, effect which is most effective when natural melatonin is not being produced—in the middle of the day—and this makes melatonin doubly useful for shift-workers and for jetlag in helping both reset the clock when timed correctly and sleep at the 'wrong' circadian phase. While melatonin and its agonists have been approved for insomnia, they are not particularly effective when taken at bedtime for non-circadian sleep disorders.

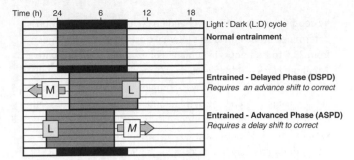

11. Treatment of circadian sleep disorders requires appropriately timed therapy to shift the timing of sleep back to the correct circadian phase. Light therapy and melatonin treatment are chronobiotic therapies whose effects depend on the circadian time of treatment (M). Treatment of delayed sleep phase disorder requires sleep to be advanced to an earlier time which can be achieved by evening melatonin treatment (M) or morning light therapy (L). Treatment of advanced sleep phase disorder requires sleep to be delayed to a later time which can be achieved with evening light exposure. Morning melatonin treatment (*M*) would also cause a phase advance but is not advised due to the sleepiness which might arise at an inappropriate time, for example while driving to work

Box 3: Living in a different time zone every day – non-24-hour sleep–wake disorder in the blind

Given that light is the most important environmental signal for setting the circadian clock, an obvious question is what happens when someone loses the ability to detect light? Unfortunately, most totally blind people, particularly those who have lost their eyes, are unable to remain synchronized to the 24-hour day and develop 'non-24-hour sleep–wake disorder' due to a mismatch between their internal clock and the 24-hour social day. This disorder is characterized by cyclic sleep problems where patients experience several weeks of good sleep followed by several weeks of poor sleep, excessive daytime sleepiness and napping, followed by good sleep again, in a never-ending cycle. The cycle duration is determined by an individual's internal clock time, which ranges from 23.6 to 25.1 hours in humans. For example, someone with a 24.5-hour clock would take 49 days (7 weeks) to complete a full 'circadian' cycle (0.5 hour/day to complete a 24.5-hour cycle). While changing sleep time by 30 minutes per day many not seem much, it soon mounts up, and soon the circadian clock is 'out of synch' with the 24-hour day, causing patients to become very sleepy during the day but awake at night. Someone with a faster clock, for example 24.1 hours, would take 241 days, or around 8 months, to go 'around the clock', and would experience 4 months of good sleep and 4 months of bad sleep each cycle. Neither the patient nor doctor may recognize this as a cyclic disorder and may inadvertently diagnose insomnia or narcolepsy given the prolonged sleep problems and excessive daytime sleepiness.

Daily melatonin treatment, taken every 24 hours in the evening, can provide a time cue to substitute for the loss of light and resynchronize the circadian clock. While all the details are not yet clear, lower doses (0.5 mg or lower) appear to best synchronize the clock but may take a few weeks to do so. Taking melatonin strictly at the same time in the evening each day, at 9 p.m., for example, would also optimize the sleepiness-inducing effects of melatonin as well as resetting the clock. As with all medications, melatonin treatment should be supervised by a doctor and non-24-hour sleep–wake disorder should be the first consideration for any totally blind individual with sleep complaints.

Parasomnias

Parasomnias are undesirable events that occur 'alongside sleep', such as sleepwalking, sleep terrors, nightmares, bedwetting ('enuresis'), sleep eating, and groaning. There are 12 categories, and they include abnormal movements, emotions, dreaming, and behaviours that occur during sleep or when waking from sleep, and they can be quite frightening, and occasionally dangerous, for the patient and bed partner. Patients may exhibit 'goal-orientated' behaviour that might make sense to them at the time but can be highly unusual by normal standards. These behaviours occur without conscious awareness and are not deliberate, a factor that often comes to the fore in legal cases if an individual is prosecuted for a physical or sexual attack during a parasomnia event.

Confusional arousals, sleepwalking, sleep terrors, nightmares, and enuresis are most common in children, although they can occur in adulthood. Confusional arousals, sleepwalking, and terrors tend to occur at the start of the night, during slow-wave sleep, with the patient exhibiting mental confusion and sometimes inappropriate behaviours. These can vary in complexity, including talking and shouting, walking, eating, and even driving, and can include physical or sexual violence. Patients may also become violent when woken and can endanger themselves, for example by trying to get through a window. During a sleep terror, the patient wakes in a physiological and behavioural state of fear, often with a terrifying scream, and sometimes accompanied by hallucinations or memories of dreams. In all three conditions, the patient may appear to be awake but often has dulled responses, sometimes having a frighteningly 'absent' or glassy look, and they usually have no memory of the events. Prior sleep deprivation is associated with these events, but other factors may affect their occurrence such as alcohol and other drug use, stress, environmental disturbance, or other medical and psychiatric conditions. Sleepwalking and confusional arousals have about the same prevalence – about 15% in children and 4% in adults, usually resolving in adolescence – and can occur together, sometimes with sleep terrors and REM behaviour disorder. Sleep terrors are less common, around 6% in children and 2% in adults.

Sleep-related eating disorder (SRED) is most often associated with sleep-walking but can occur with other sleep disorders. It occurs predominantly in young adult females with a history of childhood sleepwalking, with up to 15% of those with eating disorders reporting sleep eating. Some hypnotic and antidepressant medications appear to increase the incidence of SRED. On its own, it is not associated with any particular sleep stage, and memory of the events can vary widely between patients. Patients target high-calorie foods, not necessarily what they usually like, and will sometimes eat unusual or raw foods, or even toxic substances. Health and safety are a concern in this group of patients due to the risk of cuts or burns while preparing food, poisoning, and the potential for weight gain and obesity.

A number of parasomnias occur primarily during REM sleep, including REM behaviour disorder, sleep paralysis, sleep-related hallucinations, nightmare disorder, and sleep-related groaning. REM behaviour disorder (RBD) is abnormal or dangerous behaviour that occurs during REM sleep, and therefore tends to occur after at least 90 minutes of sleep. It affects less than 1% of the population. Usually, the normal muscle atonia characteristic of REM sleep prevents movement (Chapter 2), but in RBD patients muscle atonia is absent. Subsequently, RBD is often associated with sleep-related injury or violence, with patients 'acting out' unpleasant or violent dreams, which they remember and describe after waking. Patients do not interact with the surrounding environment and usually keep their eyes closed while expressing a wide range of physical behaviours such as talking, shouting, crawling, running, kicking, slapping, and leaping out of bed, which is why they are often injured. They do not perform the more automated behaviours seen in sleepwalking such as eating, drinking, and urinating. RBD is more common in males and generally occurs in the over 50s, and is associated with periodic limb movement disorder (see below), and neurological disorders such as Parkinson's disease, narcolepsy, multiple system atrophy, and stroke, and Tourette's syndrome and autism in children. It may also be associated with certain antidepressant medications.

Another REM-associated parasomnia is sleep paralysis, in which patients report temporarily not being able to move when falling asleep or when waking from sleep for up to several minutes, and this may be accompanied by visual or auditory hallucinations (termed 'hypnagogic hallucinations' at the start of sleep, and 'hypnopompic hallucinations' if waking up). This frightening experience is quite common, with as many as 40% of adults suffering it occasionally, and it is caused by a dissociation of REM activity and sleep so that the muscle atonia that occurs during REM sleep 'leaks' temporarily into wakefulness while falling asleep or after waking up. The sleep-related hallucinations may also occur without paralysis.

Sleep groaning also usually occurs during REM but is rare and does not appear to cause major sleep or health problems.

Nightmare disorder is a common type of parasomnia and is the occurrence of repeated violent, frightening, and emotional nightmares, usually during REM sleep although sometimes during NREM too. The disorder is often associated with stress, including acute stressful events or post-traumatic stress disorder, and is reported more in females. Some medications can increase the risk of nightmares, including some antidepressants and antihypertension drugs. Patients often wake after the nightmare and may avoid going back to sleep, inducing sleep deprivation, which can then make the problem worse. Addressing the underlying anxiety may help to reduce the occurrence of nightmares.

Sleep-related movement disorders

Restless legs syndrome (RLS) is characterized by an overwhelming urge to move the legs during periods of rest or inactivity and may affect as much as 10% of the population. Leg discomfort or pain is relieved by moving the legs or walking. Most people who report RLS may experience period limb movements during sleep (PLMS) and some during wakefulness (PLMW), particularly when trying to fall asleep. RLS can occur in all ages and is up to twice as common in women compared to men, with the risk increased by pregnancy. RLS is associated with disturbed sleep, daytime fatigue, and impaired quality of life. It can be caused by iron deficiency, which may also lead to dopamine abnormalities. Intravenous administration of iron or treatment with dopamine-receptor agonists can be highly effective.

Periodic limb movement disorder is the occurrence of rhythmic, repetitive period limb movements during sleep (PLMS), generally NREM sleep, which may not wake the patient (though it often disturbs the bed partner) but results in disturbed, unsatisfying sleep and daytime fatigue. The lower leg is mostly affected, with extension of the big toe and ankle, knee or hip movement, and repetitive leg muscle contractions, lasting 0.5–5 seconds each, that can be observed on an EMG. A PLMS Index of 5 or more events per hour plus daytime sleepiness symptoms is usually diagnostic. About one-third of over-60s have the problem, and up to 15% of insomnia patients. Most RLS patients have PLMS, as do those with REM behaviour disorder and narcolepsy. PLMS can also occur in neurological disorders that are associated with dopamine impairment such as Parkinson's disease and attention deficit hyperactivity disorder (ADHD). PLMD is not the same as the quick 'start' or hypnic jerks that people sometimes experience as they fall asleep – these tend to be shorter and are not rhythmic events.

This chapter can only provide a very broad overview of the major sleep disorders; those who wish to understand more about the causes, consequences, and treatment of the wide range of sleep problems that people can experience are directed to the Further reading section.

Chapter 7
Sleep and health

We can ask how sleep relates to health in two different ways. In the previous chapter, we examined how having a clinical sleep disorder affects your health and increases the risk of other diseases. In this chapter, we address the question of what happens to those who do not get enough sleep or suffer disrupted sleep. Studies of how sleep and disease are related are best examined by large-scale population-based research termed epidemiology. Epidemiologists take several different methodological approaches which give varying degrees of confidence in the strength of the association between an exposure (for example, sleep duration) and disease. The most robust studies follow people over a long time, maybe even a lifetime, to see how their behaviours affect the incidence of disease. Shorter studies, for example surveying a cross-section of society, can indicate disease prevalence but can only show associations between sleep and disease, not cause and effect. Both approaches have been taken with respect to sleep, and are reviewed in this chapter.

Large-scale studies examining the relationship between sleep and disease have only recently been undertaken but are showing remarkable, and sobering, connections. For example, shortened or reduced sleep duration is associated with an increased risk of a number of serious diseases including cardiovascular disease, diabetes, and certain types of cancer (Table 4). There also appears to be a close link between sleep and mental health, as outlined in the second half of this chapter.

Why didn't we appreciate these links until recently? The answer to this question is complex but a partial explanation is that sleep has never been considered sufficiently important as a subject of research in public health studies. Society in general has a broadly dismissive attitude towards sleep – how many times do we hear that 'sleep is for wimps!' or 'you can sleep when you're dead'? Although societal attitudes towards sleep are often unhelpful (see Chapter 8), powerful associations are now being established between sleep and disease. Indeed, sleep measures should become a vital part of public health research,

Table 4. Some consequences of sleep deficiency and circadian rhythm disruption

• Drowsiness, microsleeps, and unintended sleep
• Changes in mood patterns
• Anxiety and depression
• Decreased motor performance
• Decreased cognitive performance
• Impairment of memory and concentration
• Poorer communication and decision-making
• Increased irritability
• Increased risk-taking
• Weight gain
• Increased risk of metabolic disorders and diabetes
• Increased risk of hypertension, stroke, and heart attack
• Increased risk of some cancers
• Impaired immune response

perhaps as important as knowledge about smoking, alcohol, diet, and exercise.

Sleep and safety

The most immediate risk of poor sleep to our health is the risk of drowsiness-related accidents and injuries. Falling asleep while driving or working when very tired dramatically increases the risk of both fatal accidents and minor slips and lapses (see Chapters 8 and 9). Often the first thing we lose when sleepy is the ability to perform simple highly learned, 'automatic' tasks that we usually take for granted, like driving. Even small changes in sleep can be problematic; the shift to daylight saving time (DST) in Spring causes the loss of an hour's sleep and this coincides with a near 20% increase in motor vehicle accidents the Monday morning after the change. While there are individual differences in how sleep deficiency affects alertness and performance, no-one is immune from its effects, and with enough sleep loss eventually everyone would become impaired. Unfortunately, our sleepy brain cannot judge our own abilities, and as a result we are sometimes blissfully, and dangerously, unaware of our impaired performance.

Sleep and heart disease

A number of major studies have addressed the link between sleep and cardiovascular disease and show quite consistent results. People who experience reduced sleep (usually 6 hours or less) are at a higher risk of having high blood pressure, stroke, and heart disease, and die more often from heart attacks, than people who report sleeping longer (usually 7–8 hours). Interestingly, the risk of a heart attack goes up by 5% in the 3 weeks after we lose an hour's sleep during the changeover to DST, but does not happen when the clocks 'fall back' in the autumn.

Many of these studies also show a 'U-shaped' relationship between sleep and disease, with poorer health outcomes in those who report sleeping longer than normal (usually 9 hours or more). One explanation for this finding is that people with chronic illnesses or poorer general health may sleep more or stay in bed longer and therefore report sleeping longer. Whether there is a health risk of 'over-sleeping' has not been established, but it is doubtful that many people would have the chance to sleep longer than necessary in our sleep-deficient society, and so people should not be concerned about sleeping too much – the bigger risk is that most of us do not get enough sleep.

How does sleep deficiency affect the heart? The mechanisms are not yet well understood, but the metabolic consequences of sleep deprivation may lead to raised levels of fat (lipids) in the blood, which over time increases the risk of heart disease. Hypertension, and subsequently the risk of stroke and cardiovascular disease, are associated with short sleep, as is increased calcification of the arteries, a known risk factor for heart attacks that leads to the formation of more blood clots. Pro-inflammatory processes, including cytokine production and blood vessel endothelial cell function, are also affected by short sleep and are a potentially important contributor to risk of heart disease. Disrupted sleep has also been shown to be associated with higher levels of C-reactive protein, a known biomarker of heart disease.

In addition to sleep itself, other factors associated with short or disordered sleep also have the potential to affect the heart. Light exposure at night elevates heart rate and so waking repeatedly at night might increase the variability in heart function at a time when, under natural conditions, bright light would never be seen. The heart also exhibits strong daily circadian rhythms; heart rate and variability in heart rate are higher in the early morning hours, particularly during REM sleep, and the ability of platelets (blood-clotting factors) to aggregate and form clots peaks during the night. These factors, along with posture changes, hormone levels, and transitioning from sleep to being awake, appear to combine and help explain the observation that the rate of heart attacks and strokes peaks in the late morning (6 a.m. to 12 p.m.). Such marked rhythms in health and the vulnerability to disease raise the possibility of 'chronopharmacology' – delivering drugs at a time that coincides with the time of greatest risk – an emerging area of medicine with enormous potential.

Sleep and metabolism

Multiple studies have shown that short or disrupted sleep is associated with weight gain, increased fat mass deposition, obesity, and diabetes, and it is now well established that restricting sleep alters our metabolism in ways that increase the risk factors for these metabolic disorders. It is interesting to note that since the 1960s, reported sleep duration has decreased while the rate of obesity has simultaneously increased, and it is tempting to speculate that chronic sleep loss has played, and will continue to play, some part in this burgeoning health epidemic.

Detailed laboratory studies have begun to explore the underlying relationships between sleep and metabolism by examining the hormonal, energy expenditure, and appetite changes that occur when research subjects are permitted different amounts of sleep. Following sleep restriction (typically 4–5 hours versus 10–12 hours per night for up to a week), insulin is less effective at lowering blood glucose (increased insulin resistance) and the ability of glucose to regulate its own levels independent of insulin also becomes impaired (decreased glucose tolerance). High circulating blood levels of glucose damage blood vessels and eventually kidney, eye, and nerve function if not properly regulated. Sleep restriction, and particularly slow-wave sleep restriction, also alters appetite, making people hungrier and leading them to eat more, especially carbohydrates. These changes occur, not because people are awake for longer and have more opportunity to eat, but because the major hormones affecting appetite and metabolism are altered.

Adipose (fat) tissue and the stomach secrete two hormones, leptin and ghrelin, respectively, which are two of the primary factors that regulate the brain centres controlling appetite. Leptin is a 'satiety' hormone – high levels of leptin inhibit feeding and reduce our appetite. Leptin is stimulated by feeding, helping us to know when we have had enough to eat, and is generally higher at night to ensure that we eat at the right time of day (see below). Ghrelin has the opposite effect – high levels stimulate our appetite, and levels increase with increasing time between meals. The ratio of these two hormones helps to regulate our appetite; after a meal, we have high leptin and low ghrelin which reduces our appetite. Sleep restriction, however, alters this balance, reducing the amount of leptin and increasing the amount of ghrelin, making us hungrier. Chronic sleep restriction is therefore likely to lead us to overeat, and to eat more carbohydrates, resulting in obesity, insulin resistance, and higher glucose levels, all of which are risk factors for type II diabetes. Indeed, epidemiological studies have shown that reported short sleepers (6 or fewer hours), or those with problems initiating or maintaining sleep, have about a 2- to 3-fold increase in diabetes risk as compared to those reporting 7–8 hours sleep per night.

While it is clear that sleep restriction plays a role in appetite regulation and metabolic function, most studies have restricted sleep by extending the day, which also means extending the duration of light exposure and altering the night duration. Sleep–wake cycles gate light exposure to the brain as we are usually exposed to light when awake and shut off most light exposure when we close our eyes to sleep. Given that humans still maintain the ability to detect changes in night duration through their melatonin rhythm (Chapter 2), some of these metabolic changes may also be due to the effects of light exposure at night directly or photoperiodic changes. Interestingly, some of the symptoms of seasonal affective disorder, the depression brought on by seasonal changes in night duration, are similar to those experienced during sleep restriction, including carbohydrate craving, appetite changes, and weight gain. The widespread use of electric lighting at night effectively consigns society to live in a never-ending metabolic summer – perhaps the increased rates of obesity are in part because we never experience a biochemical winter to use up the fat stores laid down earlier in the year. Disruption of seasonal cycles has never been studied in humans but, after tens of thousands of years of evolution in a natural light–dark cycle, it is difficult to imagine that there will not be any adverse effects.

Like many other physiological and biochemical processes, our metabolism also exhibits a distinct daily pattern; a meal eaten at 1:30 a.m. will result in higher blood levels of glucose, insulin, and fats for several hours after the meal as compared to eating the same meal at 1:30 p.m. The size of the effect is so large in some people that their blood glucose levels look like those of a diabetic, simply by eating at night. As a diurnal (day-active) animal, humans have evolved to metabolize food optimally during the daytime, and so eating at night results in far less efficient processing. This is a chronic problem in shift-workers and partly underlies the increased risk of diabetes and heart disease that they experience (Chapter 9). Even in non-shift-workers, however, eating later will likely lead to similar problems – the northern British tradition of having the largest meal in the middle of the day ('dinner' time) with a smaller 'tea' in the early evening makes the most sense in this context, although those who keep a Mediterranean 'siesta' lifestyle, including a late evening meal, may disagree.

Sleep and immune function

Two groups of people were immunized against the influenza virus while keeping two different sleep schedules; the group who were allowed to sleep only 4 hours per night when given the jab had less than half the level of protective antibody to the virus than the group who slept their usual 7.5–8.5 hours per night. Similar results have been shown for the antibody response to a hepatitis A vaccination which is blunted in those who are sleep-deprived. Fatigue and sleepiness are often symptoms associated with inflammatory disorders, and people tend to sleep more if they become ill. The role of sleep in immune function, and the effect of the immune system on sleep, are thus beginning to be explored. Sleep restriction appears to increase levels of circulating cytokines such as interleukin 6 (IL-6) and tumour necrosis factor α (TNF-α) and other inflammatory markers such as high-sensitivity C-reactive protein (hs-CRP), factors that increase the risk of cardiovascular disease and diabetes.

The role of sleep as a potential intervention to facilitate healing has not been explored systematically, but may have great potential. The sleeping environment provided in hospitals, for example, is usually very poor, with frequent disturbance due to noise from other patients, late night or early morning scheduling of procedures and rounds which curtail time for sleep, weak light–dark cycles, and a general failure to prioritize patient sleep in the day-to-day running of the modern hospital. Several small studies suggest that access to daylight can reduce stress and use of pain medication post-surgery, and reduce the length of patient stay. Given our improved understanding of the connections between immune function and sleep, greater focus on patient sleep may have benefits on the extent and rate of their recovery. Greater focus on the sleep and alertness of healthcare providers will also benefit patient care, as discussed in Chapter 9.

Sleep and cancer

Most work concerning sleep disruption and cancer has focused on the risk of cancer in shift-workers. As reviewed in Chapter 9, shift-workers, who experience both extreme circadian rhythm disruption and sleep disruption, have around a 50% increased risk of breast and prostate cancer compared to women and men who have not worked shifts. While the mechanistic links between sleep disruption and cancer remain unclear, several possibilities have been proposed, including (i) disruption of immune function; (ii) exposure to light at night causing lower melatonin levels; (iii) disturbance of cell cycle rhythms; (iv) sleep or circadian- controlled alterations in multiple hormonal and metabolic systems.

Sleep, mental health, and neurodegenerative disease

The association between sleep disruption and overall brain function has a long history. Emil Kraepelin, one of the founders of modern psychiatry, noted in his first textbook, of 1883, that abnormal sleep patterns and poor mental health occur together. Despite this recognized connection, cause and effect have been much debated without reaching any firm conclusions. The recent advances in our understanding of the neural basis of sleep and circadian rhythm generation have allowed both a re-evaluation of these connections and the understanding of the importance of sleep to the healthy brain. A new conceptual framework is emerging which can be summarized as follows.

At the core of any psychiatric disorder or neurodegenerative disease will be an abnormality in neurotransmitter signalling. As sleep and circadian timing systems utilize a large number of neurotransmitters (Chapter 3), it should be no surprise that sleep complaints are reported in more than 80% of patients with either depression or schizophrenia, and that sleep abnormalities are common in both Alzheimer's disease and Parkinson's disease patients. Disruption of sleep and circadian rhythms will in turn have widespread effects, ranging across all aspects of neural and neuroendocrine function including impaired cognition, emotions, metabolic abnormalities, reduced immunity, and elevated risks of cancer and coronary heart disease. A spectrum of clinical pathologies, matching those reported for sleep disruption (Table 4), are also routinely reported as occurring with brain disorders but are rarely linked to the disruption in sleep.

Furthermore, sleep and circadian rhythm disruption will lead to abnormal light exposure and atypical patterns of social behaviour, further destabilizing normal physiology and exacerbating an abnormal pattern of neurotransmitter release within the brain. In turn, this could lead to a state of internal desynchronization of numerous hormonal and behavioural rhythms. Add to this the impact of medication (e.g. the use of antipsychotics or cholinesterase inhibitors) and the possibility of addiction and substance abuse, and the net result is the potentially significant disruption of multiple neural and neuroendocrine pathways. Indeed, such sets of interacting factors could explain the variable nature of sleep disruptions observed in psychiatric disorders and neurodegenerative disease, with relatively small changes in the environment potentially amplifying an individual's vulnerability to illness. This discussion highlights the difficulty of assigning simple 'cause and effect' interpretations to any abnormal sleep phenotype in individuals with a mental health condition or neurodegenerative disease.

Abnormalities in sleep timing and sleep EEG are recognized as common co-morbid problems in numerous psychiatric disorders. Indeed, changes in sleep behaviour are listed as a key criterion for the diagnosis of affective (mood) disorders in current classification schemes of mental disorders (such as the *Diagnostic and Statistical Manual of Mental Disorders* IV-*Text Revision*, DSM- IV-TR). Up to 90% of patients suffering from an acute depressive episode report simultaneous changes in their sleep profile that are usually described as difficulties falling to sleep and maintaining sleep during the night. Interestingly, persistent insomnia increases the risk of relapse into a new depressive episode, and increased sleep disruption, as in mothers after childbirth, raises the risk of post-partum depression, with poorer sleep quality correlating with more severe depression. Some of the tricyclic antidepressants (e.g. amitriptyline, imipramine, clomipramine) and non-tricyclic antidepressants (e.g. trazodone or mirtazapine) have very pronounced sedative effects, and are commonly used as sleeping agents in non-depressed individuals. As a result, part of the efficacy of some antidepressants may be by their direct action on sleep.

Bipolar disorder is a broad term for illnesses ranging from major or minor depression to major or minor mood elevation (mania and hypomania) and from low-grade mood cycling to full psychosis. It is clear that irregular sleep timing and a reduction in total sleep time is an important factor in the incidence of manic episodes, and in predisposed individuals disruption of their 24-hour sleep–wake cycle, shortened sleep, or travel across multiple time zones seems to act as an important trigger for a relapse (77% of patients) into mania. As a result, treatment therapies frequently involve regimes that stabilize the schedule and behaviour and permit adequate sleep, although well-tested consistent clinical guidelines for such therapies are lacking.

Sleep in patients with alcohol problems is disturbed both on drinking and non-drinking nights. During periods of heavy drinking, and up to two years after stopping, sleep shows reduced SWS states, suppressed REM sleep, fragmented sleep during the second half of the night, and shortened overall sleep duration. Rates of insomnia in alcoholics are reported to be between 40% and 70%.

Sleep disorders are also reported in 30–80% of schizophrenia patients and are one of the most common symptoms of the disorder. Patients with schizophrenia show poor sleep and score badly on many quality-of-life assessments, and an improvement in sleep is one of the highest priorities in their treatment. Improvement of sleep quality in schizophrenia is frequently correlated with an improvement in negative symptoms. The relationship between disrupted sleep and various anxiety-related disorders is also well recognized, and in this case, cause and effect is even more difficult to untangle. For example, insomnia predisposes individuals to anxiety, which precipitates sleep disruption that in turn increases the likelihood of panic (Chapter 6). Conversely, there is evidence that sleep problems precede conditions such as anxiety and depression.

Abnormal sleep is also closely associated with neurodegenerative disease. As with mental health, the sleep pattern is variable and the specific mechanistic connections remain poorly defined. Unsurprisingly, when neurodegenerative disease affects the brain structures and neurotransmitters involved in sleep and circadian rhythms (Chapter 3), sleep disruption is the result. Neurodegenerative disease is usually progressive and irreversible, but the treatment of sleep–wake and rest–activity abnormalities in these pathologies is emerging as a possible approach to improve the overall condition and quality of life of patients, and in some cases may even slow the progression of physical and mental decline. In Alzheimer's disease, for example, fragmented nighttime sleep is highly debilitating to both patients and caregivers and is a primary reason for transferring patients into a nursing home. A notable feature of Alzheimer's disease is 'sundowning', or a tendency to be confused and agitated in the late afternoon and evening. This might be related to mental and physical exhaustion at the end of the day, but reduced light at this time of day may also contribute to impaired levels of cognitive alertness, particularly in patients in care homes, where lighting is often poor (Chapter 5).

The earliest description of the 'shaking palsy' (Parkinson's disease) by James Parkinson included a reference to disturbed sleep. Both nighttime sleep disturbances and daytime sleepiness occur in Parkinson's disease, and it has been estimated that 80–90% of Parkinson's disease patients have a sleep disorder which affects their ability to fall asleep and stay asleep, their dreams, motor activity during sleep, and daytime sleepiness. Neuronal cell loss occurs in the substantia nigra in the brain leading to dopamine deficiency, and also occurs within those brainstem nuclei critical for the regulation of sleep-wake states (Chapter 3). Degeneration of these nuclei leads to disruption of basic REM and NREM sleep architecture. Substantial evidence suggests that abnormal REM sleep behaviour precedes Parkinsonism and dementia by several years and therefore might provide a useful marker during the early phase of Parkinson's disease and a possibility for early intervention.

Huntington's disease patients also show progressive abnormalities in sleep and circadian behaviour which is associated with atrophy of key brain structures involved in the regulation of sleep such as the brainstem and lateral hypothalamus.

Patients with multiple sclerosis (MS) and demyelination of neuronal pathways show disrupted nighttime sleep and daytime sleepiness, which is frequently correlated with increased levels of pain, fatigue, and depression. Given the complex interactions of the multiple neuronal systems involved in sleep generation and sleep–wake control, demyelination in one or more of these neuronal systems could profoundly affect sleep and arousal in MS.

In view of the discussion above, the stabilization of the sleep and circadian systems might be expected to have a positive effect on both quality of life and disease symptoms in psychiatric illness and neurodegenerative disease. Evidence is emerging that such a stabilization is beneficial. For example, bright-light phototherapy has been used as an entrainment signal for the circadian system and has been shown to alleviate some of the symptoms of several mood disorders including unipolar depression and bipolar depression, although it can induce mania in some bipolar patients. Daily melatonin treatment can also act to entrain the circadian system. In combination with light or melatonin, social cues can also be useful in regulating the circadian/sleep system. Stabilizing activities such as exercise and meals can influence daily patterns of light exposure and modify the timing of behaviour by associative learning and reinforcement, and could prove valuable when incorporated into cognitive behavioural therapy paradigms to treat sleep disorders (Chapter 6).

It is important to keep in mind that many of the associations between sleep and health discussed above are indeed just that at this point in time – an association. Most studies to date have used techniques that do not permit cause to be determined. While clinical trials will be useful in establishing cause and effect of sleep disruption on short-term health risks, more accurate measurements of sleep, in large populations followed over many years, are needed to determine whether sleep has life-long small effects on long-term health outcomes. It is already clear, however, that sleep is an essential behaviour and should be considered one of the key pillars of good health, along with diet and exercise, and should therefore be elevated in our list of health priorities.

Chapter 8
Sleep and society

Society plays an enormous role in shaping our attitudes towards sleep, which in turn affects how much sleep we get. Sleep also has a major impact upon society, influencing childhood learning and development, affecting workplace safety and efficiency, and driving multi-billion-pound industries aimed at helping us get better sleep or counteracting inadequate sleep. Sleepiness and sleep disorders cost the economy billions of pounds each year in days off, lost time, inefficient work, and accidents, yet the machismo associated with short sleep and long work hours is pervasive. Society glorifies 'driven' individuals who succeed on apparently little sleep, whereas those who prioritize sleep are viewed as weak and not having the 'right stuff'. Some professions even demand excessive sleep deprivation as part of the job or a 'rite of passage'. These attitudes are outdated and ultimately counterproductive, however, both individually and across a profession, as failing to get sufficient sleep has major consequences for safety, productivity, and health.

Sleep and driving

Drowsy-driving kills or seriously injures twice as many people each year on Britain's roads as drug use, and about one-third of the number of people killed by drunk-driving. Drowsiness is the cause of about one-fifth of all accidents on major roads according to government figures. These numbers are likely to be an underestimate, however, as drowsy-driving accidents are difficult to detect and can often be miscategorized. For example, in accidents involving alcohol or drugs, sleepiness is also a major factor in the cause. Slower reaction times, poor decision-making, failure to look properly, carelessness, distraction, and other accident categorizations are also more likely when sleepy. Society is not completely unaware of the problem – in the UK, for example, drivers see 'Tiredness Can Kill' road-signs on the motorway and are told how to use naps and caffeine effectively if too tired to drive. While helpful, simply raising awareness may not be enough, and at least 500, and perhaps as many as 3,500, people are needlessly killed or seriously injured because of drowsy drivers on Britain's roads each year, with hundreds of thousands more worldwide.

Drowsy-driving accidents are of greatest concern in young people, who account for a disproportionately high number of them. The rate of accidents peaks at night in all drivers when the circadian rhythm in sleepiness is at its highest, but young people are likely to be more sleep-deprived and are less able to withstand a lack of sleep than older drivers, at least in laboratory tests. This lethal combination had led many US states to develop curfews banning new drivers from driving unaccompanied late at night (e.g. 0:30 to 5:00 a.m.) to counter the risk of falling asleep at the wheel, as well as mitigating novice drivers' inexperience, risk-taking behaviour, and drink and drug use.

So why does society not take drowsy-driving seriously? We certainly recognize the problem, given the range of behaviours that people employ to stay awake, like chewing gum, fresh air, loud music, talking to someone on the phone, or more extreme solutions like a drawing-pin bracelet. People often realize that they are dangerously sleepy but prefer to do anything except address the real cause – the lack of sleep. There are sometimes complex reasons for staying awake a long time and then driving, such as a financial necessity to work long hours or take on multiple jobs, or while caring for children or elderly relatives. Other factors, such as family commitments, hobbies, social life, or simply sitting and reading a book, squeeze the limited time available for sleep and pressure people into driving while sleepy. Many people also choose to 'burn the candle at both ends' and disregard the risks, and the low probability of being caught reinforces this attitude – there is no roadside breathalyser or blood-test for sleepiness (although much effort is going into to finding one). Assigning sleepiness as the cause of an accident is also difficult for several reasons. First, our ability to judge our own level of impairment is compromised by sleepiness; much like a drunk brain, the sleepy brain cannot evaluate itself and often underestimates how sleepy we are. Objective signs of unsafe levels of sleepiness, like yawning and slower blinks, are often ignored. Second, catastrophic sleepiness can come on immediately and without warning, so an individual may not recall falling asleep, or even being sleepy, before the accident – it takes only a few seconds of sleepiness to career off the road. Sleepiness is not high on the list of potential causes in the accident report, with a greater likelihood that another easier-to-detect reason will be listed. There are tell-tale signs of drowsy-driving accidents – a gradual veering off the road without braking, or single-vehicle accidents occurring at night in otherwise good conditions, for example – but sleepiness as a cause of accidents is difficult to prove without an individual's sleep history for the past few days. We do leave a trail of wakefulness in the electronic age, however, with telephone, internet, GPS, and credit card records all able to reveal our sleep–wake state, but even with these tools, proving sleepiness immediately prior to an accident is difficult.

As was the case for drunk-driving, a shift in society's attitude to drowsy-driving is needed in order to make any substantial gains. The comparison to drunk-driving is a real one; 24 hours of continuous wakefulness induces a performance impairment equivalent to being legally drunk (Figure 12). Sleepy-driving is scoffed at today in the way that drunk-driving was 30 years ago, and the scorn now reserved for those drunk behind the wheel must extend to those who are sleepy behind the wheel. We demand that those driving planes, trains, and automobiles do so sober and are fit for duty (although sadly, there are plenty of examples of fatigued pilots, train drivers, bus drivers, and many others having catastrophic fall-asleep crashes), and society should demand the same responsibility towards sleep. A major step towards this aim would be for the public to understand the consequences of 'second-hand sleepiness' in the same terms as is now understood for 'second-hand smoking'. While it may be an individual choice to increase the risk of killing yourself through your own drowsy-driving, it is not acceptable to increase the risk of killing or injuring others. Obtaining adequate sleep is an individual's personal responsibility and a requirement before driving any vehicle, and failure to do so is a preventable and unacceptable crime.

Awareness of the risks, and ways to prevent them, are key in this effort. This might mean that obese individuals, who have a very high risk of obstructive sleep apnoea, have to reduce their risk of sleepiness by getting treatment and losing weight in order to be allowed to drive cars, trucks, or the school bus; mothers who shuttle their children around in 'four-by-fours' to keep their own children safe must not drive if sleepy and risk killing other mothers' children; doctors who we consider are no longer safe to work after 13 hours should not be considered safe to drive home afterwards. These are difficult questions for society to face but have serious consequences and warrant our attention. Use of public transport (provided the drivers are properly slept), living closer to school and work, actively planning sleep opportunities ahead of time, and overall prioritization of sleep, need to be considered in the same way as we plan ahead so we are not drunk when we drive to work or drop the children off at school.

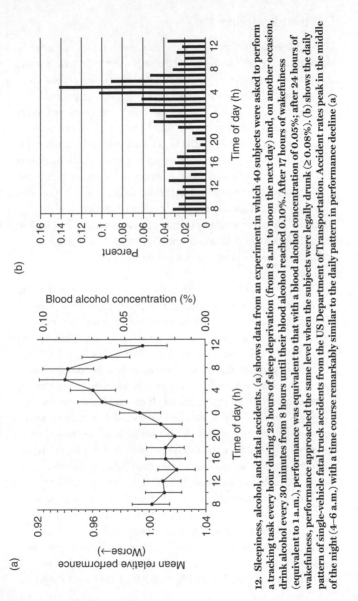

12. **Sleepiness, alcohol, and fatal accidents.** (a) shows data from an experiment in which 40 subjects were asked to perform a tracking task every hour during 28 hours of sleep deprivation (from 8 a.m. to noon the next day) and, on another occasion, drink alcohol every 30 minutes from 8 hours until their blood alcohol reached 0.10%. After 17 hours of wakefulness (equivalent to 1 a.m.), performance was equivalent to that with a blood alcohol concentration of 0.05%; after 24 hours of wakefulness, performance approached the same level when the subjects were legally drunk (≥ 0.08%). (b) shows the daily pattern of single-vehicle fatal truck accidents from the US Department of Transportation. Accident rates peak in the middle of the night (4–6 a.m.) with a time course remarkably similar to the daily pattern in performance decline (a)

Sleep and caffeine

One of the reasons that society can function without sufficient sleep is that we self-medicate. Caffeine is a central nervous system stimulant that blocks the effects of adenosine which builds up during wakefulness as a by-product of using up our internal energy stores (Chapter 3). It is an extremely valuable commodity, with an annual global market of $22 billion, supporting as many as 75 million livelihoods. Caffeine is found primarily in tea, coffee, and soft drinks (50–80 milligrams per cup or can), although it is also found in chocolate, with other drugs to increase effectiveness, or in pill form over-the-counter. It is available in ever higher doses in energy drinks (sometimes with alcohol), and boutique drinks, countering a society-wide epidemic of sleepiness and insufficient sleep. The average Briton consumes about 300 milligrams of caffeine per day, or over 2 grams per week.

Caffeine's pharmacological effects include improved reaction time and alertness but also increased blood pressure, heart rate, and body temperature. Its effects on sleep, even if taken in the morning, include longer sleep latency, reduced sleep duration, and suppression of slow-wave 'deep' sleep. At high levels (> 300 milligrams acute dose, or 500–600 milligrams per day), it can induce jitteriness and muscle twitches, headaches, anxiety, and heart palpitations, and with chronic high use, can also cause ulcers and acid reflux disease and lead to caffeine-induced anxiety and sleep disorders. Users develop tolerance, with ever-higher doses needed to induce the same response, and it is therefore an addictive drug. When stopped, users experience withdrawal symptoms including headaches, nausea, fatigue, irritability, trembling, and insomnia for up to 5 days. The drug has a long 'half-life' – about 5 hours, and longer under some circumstances – meaning that it takes about 5 hours to metabolize half of the circulating amount. This means that if someone has a coffee or soda containing 100 milligrams of caffeine at 10 a.m. in the morning, there are still 25 milligrams left in the body by 8 p.m. at night, and about 12.5 milligrams at bedtime, which causes measureable disruption of sleep. In practice, people use much higher amounts, and use it late into the day, even after dinner, inducing poor-quality sleep (even in those who swear that caffeine does not affect them). Individual sensitivities to caffeine are apparent due to tolerance and in part to our genes – differences in the adenosine A2A receptor gene are associated with caffeine sensitivity and the degree of sleep disturbance when using caffeine, possibly contributing to the high prevalence of insomnia.

In an ideal world, we would all get sufficient sleep and not need any caffeine, but if we must in order to stay safe, the trick is to use it 'little and often' to maintain alertness with minimum caffeine intake, and to stop using it as long as possible before bedtime. The alerting benefits can be achieved at relatively modest doses (0.3 mg/kg/hour – about 20 mg/hour in a 70-kg person), which is equivalent to 1 cup of normal tea, weak coffee, or soda approximately every 2 hours. Higher caffeine intake is unnecessary, and consuming large quantities at the start of the day or workshift is unhelpful as caffeine levels will decline as sleepiness increases through the day. Stopping caffeine use at least 5 hours, and ideally 10 hours, before trying to sleep is also advisable.

Caffeine is more powerful in children due to their smaller size and less frequent exposure and they should avoid it. Preventing caffeine intake is difficult, however, as parents are competing against powerful and wealthy advertising campaigns marketed specifically to children and young adults for caffeine-containing sodas, iced-teas, and chocolate, high-end speciality teas and coffees, and lifestyle-enhancing energy drinks, which are particularly attractive to teens and young adults. While attention has been paid to limiting access to these products in schools to try and reduce sugar intake, their potentially harmful effects on sleep have not yet been addressed. Limiting or banning access to such drinks in schools and in the home in an attempt to reduce childhood obesity would have an additional benefit in improving children's sleep, which might in turn further reduce their risk of obesity, and would address both health issues in a substantial way – a 'win-win' that society should bravely embrace.

Sleep and school

It is no surprise that teenagers and young adults use caffeine when we consider how the odds are stacked up against them getting sufficient sleep. As outlined in Chapter 5, adolescents experience a delay in their circadian clocks that drives them to sleep and wake later than younger children and adults and leads to chronic sleep deprivation, particularly on school days. Early school start times affect adolescent sleep in two ways. First, the delay in the clock prevents teenagers from going to sleep early and therefore prevents them from getting the 8–9 hours of sleep per night that they need. Second, the delay in the clock also means that requiring teenagers to get up for school at 6 or 7 a.m. is the equivalent of asking adults to wake up at 3 or 4 a.m. in the morning. Rising at this time causes severe sleep inertia and coincides with the circadian dip in mood and cognition. Short sleep is also associated with increased classroom sleepiness, lower grades, and poorer mood and behaviour, and is likely to increase hyperactivity, irritability, or aggression. Short sleep may also be contributing to increases in childhood obesity rates (see Chapter 5) and may be associated with more serious psychological disorders such as depression. A recent study showed that if parents permit late bedtimes (midnight or later), their children have an increased risk of depression and suicidal ideation.

A simple solution, although not simple to implement, is to delay school, college, and university start times, allowing students to sleep longer and wake at a more appropriate circadian phase. It has been known for more than a decade that later school start times are associated with longer sleep, better alertness and concentration, and better grades. Class times are currently designed for adults, requiring children to truncate their sleep every day, which undoubtedly has a negative impact on their educational achievement by impairing vigilance and memory (Box 4). In the US, studies have shown that delaying school start times by as little as 30–90 minutes can improve student sleep duration and quality, academic performance, absenteeism and lateness rates, mood, alertness, and health. A one-hour change was also shown to reduce the rate of automobile crashes in 17–18-year-olds by 17%. Contrary to many expectations, later school start times do not lead to later bedtimes – bedtime remains constant and sleep duration increases – reflecting the biological basis of the problem.

While the complexity of changing school start times appears overwhelming, with factors such as curriculum targets, parental work times, school transport, teaching hours, and extracurricular programmes to be considered, these should be secondary to the

Box 4: Sleep and learning

We know from personal experience that 'sleeping on it' often helps to solve a problem. Recent research is beginning to unravel why. If subjects are taught a simple learning task, such as a 'finger-tapping' sequence, sleeping the night after learning the task somehow imprints it into memory and the subjects get better at the task. Failure to sleep after being taught the task, however, prevents any subsequent improvement in performance, even after sleeping normally for several nights. It is as if by missing sleep after learning, the brain misses the opportunity to solidify what has been learned. Similar studies have shown that developing 'insight' or higher-level learning also depends on sleep, with different types of learning dependent on different stages of sleep. Regularity and stability of sleep also seem to be important in retaining information. Obviously, these findings have important consequences for childhood learning, especially if children's sleep is curtailed on school nights.

priority of providing children with the best possible educational opportunities. Immediate advances in educational attainment could be achieved with a relatively simple step that does not require new teaching methods, new testing, or additional funds. Good policies should be based on good evidence, and the data show that children are placed at an enormous disadvantage by being asked to keep adult hours.

Sleep and work

A major societal factor affecting sleep in adults is, of course, work. Longer work hours are associated with shorter sleep and increased risk of accident and injury, and accident risk increases with increased time on the job; the risk of accident during the twelfth hour of work is more than double the risk in the first hour (Figure 13). Night work is also inherently more dangerous than day shifts (Chapter 9). While sleep is not the only factor influencing workplace injury and accident, it is a major and often manageable component of risk, and through work-hour limits and fatigue-management programmes, large gains in workplace safety and efficiency can be achieved.

One powerful countermeasure to workplace sleepiness is to permit and schedule naps. A short 'power' nap, 10–30 minutes in duration, has been shown to improve alertness and performance for up to 2–3 hours after the nap. Longer naps, 30 minutes or more, have longer-lasting effects but can also induce sleep inertia immediately after the nap, introducing a new hazard. Sleep inertia can be countered by taking caffeine prior to the nap, however, which takes about 20 minutes to kick in and is therefore 'ready' to counter the sleepiness upon waking. (The same approach can be taken to reduce sleepiness temporarily when driving.) Introduction of protected time for short naps in the workplace should be considered to improve performance and safety at little or no cost, and the increased productivity after the nap outweighs the time used napping.

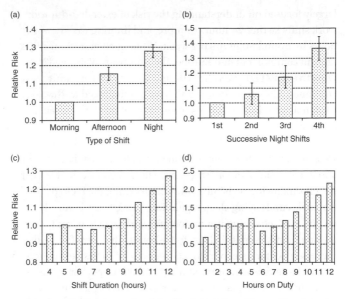

13. Factors that increase the risk of industrial accidents. Consistent with the circadian rhythm in sleepiness, the risk of accidents is highest for night shifts as compared to afternoon or morning shifts (a). Risk increases with the number of consecutive night shifts (b), in part due to the build-up of chronic sleep deficiency when the shift-worker fails to get sufficient sleep during the daytime between shifts. Accident risk increases with scheduled shift duration, with 12-hour shifts having nearly 30% higher risk than 8-hour shifts (c). Finally, accident risk increases with hours on duty, with the 10th hour of work nearly doubling the risk of an accident as compared to the first 8 hours on duty, and the 12th hour more than doubles this risk. Equivalent data are not available for shifts longer than 12 hours, but such extended shifts are certainly liable to increase accident risk even further

Is there any evidence that work-hour limits improve sleep and workplace performance? Ironically, the most robust evidence on the dangers of inadequate sleep on health comes from studies of junior doctors, driven by concerns about how patient safety is affected by doctors' long work hours. In the US, this effort has largely focused on understanding the risk of extended-duration work shifts lasting 24 hours or more, and limiting weekly work hours to around 80 hours per week. While such marathon shifts are still common outside Europe, the European Working Time Directive (EWTD) and other UK and EU regulations limit continuous duty to 13 hours, and have gradually reduced weekly work hours for junior doctors from 72 to 48 hours per week, on average.

Despite the differing situations, measurable gains in patient safety and doctors' sleep and alertness have been demonstrated in both systems following revision of work hours using the biological principles underlying sleep regulation. In a US randomized clinical trial, changing junior doctors' work schedule from 24-hour shifts every third day to 16-hour shifts every fourth day increased doctors' sleep from 6.6 hours to 7.4 hours per night, and reduced attentional failures at night by half. Importantly, there were 36% more serious medical errors when doctors worked 24-hour shifts as compared to when the same doctors worked 16-hour shifts, including nearly 6 times as many serious diagnostic errors and 21% more medication errors. In a similar UK study, doctors' hours were reduced from an average of 52 to 43 hours per week (and from a maximum of 77 to 60 hours per week), and continuous duty was limited to 12 hours maximum. The pattern of shifts was also changed; only 2–3 consecutive night shifts were permitted, versus 7 in the traditional system, and shift changes were more gradual. Doctors' sleep increased following the intervention, particularly after evening and night shifts, and medical error rates fell by 33% overall. These studies show that large gains in patient safety can be obtained, almost literally overnight, if doctors' hours are planned in accordance with the biology of sleep, and they illustrate that high levels of motivation and training cannot override the effects of sleep loss.

Unfortunately, many professions, including the medical profession, are pushing for longer shifts. While often presented as a way of getting the work done quickly, leaving more time for family and improving quality of life, the reality is that longer shifts are desired so that individuals can work second jobs and earn more money, further increasing weekly work hours and the risk of drowsy-driving or being sleepy on the job. While society expects 24/7 services, there are good and bad ways to achieve these aims, and the public should realize the unintended consequences of permitting such shifts, particularly how it places them at risk through 'second-hand sleepiness' (Chapter 9).

The impact of sleep disruption is not limited to clinicians and caregivers. Patient sleep in hospitals is notoriously poor, and as poor and shortened sleep can affect immune function and is closely associated with an increased risk of disease (see Chapter 6), it is surprising that more efforts have not been taken to improve the sleep environment in hospitals. Even small improvements could have beneficial effects on patient recovery and experience. Simple approaches could include considering sleep when scheduling events – many patients are woken unnecessarily early, for example. A quiet, dim rest period during the day could allow patients to take a nap. Reconsidering the light, noise, and temperature environment at night to permit better-quality sleep, and ensuring patients are exposed to a robust light–dark cycle is likely to improve sleep and wake quality (see Chapter 5) – access to good daytime lighting has been shown to affect patient recovery rates and outcomes. These considerations extend to other institutions such as care homes, prisons, and boarding schools.

Sleep and society

Many 'societal' factors affect our sleep, including children, pets, noise pollution, light pollution, temperature, bed type, pain, daylight saving time, gender, bed partner, diurnal preference, socioeconomic status, work, hobbies, alcohol, drugs and medications, exercise, television, radio, computers, telephones – the list goes on and on. Some of these factors can be relatively simple to deal with on an individual level – using black-out curtains or wearing an eye-mask, using ear-plugs, wearing bedsocks, taking the TV, radio, computer, telephone, and pets out of the bedroom, drinking less alcohol, exercising earlier, and going to bed earlier. There is no shame in sleeping in separate beds, or even separate rooms, if it means better sleep.

Some factors require broader more difficult solutions and require better education of the public and a political desire to make changes. For example, light pollution has potentially damaging effects on human sleep and health, and reducing light pollution would also have enormous benefits for energy conservation, improve the survival of many other species, and allow us to see the full glory of the night sky. There are straightforward solutions including simply pointing lamps downwards, not up, using timers and motion-sensors, using the right type and power of lamp, or even just turning the lights off when not needed. Requiring companies to reduce their noise pollution, or further limiting times when noisy work can start and stop, would have minimal impact on their work but great benefits for society. Greater emphasis on protecting sleep is required, and sometimes public health may need to be conserved over the individual; for example, how many people's sleep is disturbed by car alarms each night, most of which go off by accident? Manufacturers could make them less sensitive to protect our sleep which may be more beneficial to society than a tiny increase in car theft. While financial gains drive a greater and greater number of night flights, is it really necessary to fly those few thousand people around when many thousands more are adversely affected by the aeroplane noise each night? After we lose an hour's sleep when converting to daylight saving time, the rate of car crashes increases by 20% and the risk of a heart attack goes up by 5% – is this worth it, compared to the gains in converting to DST?

Do we really need to light vast acreages of car parks, industrial parks, office buildings, and back gardens when the security benefits are minimal? Do we really need 24-hour supermarkets? Do we really need 24-hour television? How did we manage before?

Part of society's failure to recognize the importance of sleep and to protect it is that the impact of poor sleep and sleep disorders is virtually untaught in medical and nursing schools. While sleep medicine is now recognized as a medical speciality in its own right in the US, this is not the case elsewhere, and healthcare providers who develop an interest in sleep are dispersed among many specialities including respiratory medicine, neurology, anaesthesiology, psychiatry, psychology, and dentistry, with inconsistencies in their training, diagnosis, and treatment of sleep problems. While some medical schools have developed courses in sleep medicine, the general level of teaching and understanding of sleep by doctors is poor, especially considering that sleep problems are one of the major complaints heard by general practitioners. We need to spend one-third of our lives asleep, yet doctors are poorly equipped to help us do so. An integrated and dedicated approach to sleep medicine training is needed given the wide impact sleep disorders have on health and society.

There are some 'societal' factors that are difficult to address. There are gender differences in how we sleep and how we perceive sleep problems (Chapter 6). A number of genes have been identified which are associated with sleep timing and sleep duration, and these intrinsic factors help to determine whether we are naturally short sleepers, or long sleepers, or prefer to wake early or go to bed late – the latter can be a problem if a couple are set at different times. The impact of children on parents' sleep is life-changing and can last for many years. There are no easy solutions to these issues, but awareness of the importance of sleep, and following your own sleep preferences where possible, may help raise the priority of sleep in your own, your family's, or your employees' lives. Meeting the challenge to prioritize sleep is integral to the success of our society and requires an educated approach to balance economic, family, and health concerns. With progressive leadership by individuals and institutions, society can undo the many misconceptions about sleep and support a more sleep-friendly lifestyle.

Chapter 9
The 24-hour society

We live increasingly in a 24-hour society – 24-hour news coverage, all-night supermarkets, continuous internet availability – all of which is chipping away at our time for sleep. With the culture of working long hours, globalization of businesses, and the ever-increasing need for overnight shift-work and flexible working hours, society seems to be conspiring to demote sleep in our list of priorities. It was not that long ago that the small number of TV channels available finished their programming at the end of the night. The national anthem was still played at the end of BBC1 programming as recently as 1997, with the announcer saying presciently on the last occasion '...instead of leaving you in the dark at closedown, we'll be joining a brand new service, BBC News 24, with through-the-night coverage and reports from around the globe. In the meantime, we're heading for some shut-eye...'. We have since been invited to shop, buy petrol, watch TV, drink in the pub, or surf the web around the clock, whether we asked for it or not. The key to all this activity is the ability to light the night, without which none of these nocturnal excursions would be possible.

The power to remove darkness was once held only by deities, but the ability to light the night fell into mortal hands at the end of the 19th century, with the development and widespread installation of electric incandescent lighting. While it was possible before this time to light the night with fire, candles, kerosene and gas lamps, a steady, reliable, and safe source of nighttime illumination was only possible using electricity and, largely through the entrepreneurial drive of Thomas Edison, spread and continues to spread, very rapidly. In the US, for example, around 300,000 general lighting service lamps were sold by 1885, which grew to nearly 90 million lamps by 1914, and 800 million lamps annually by 1945. Today, approximately 2 billion bulbs are sold each year in the US, and nearly one-quarter of all electricity sold is used for lighting. These advances revolutionized society and made it possible to consider 24-hour-a-day services.

Innovations in jet travel created similarly unnatural light exposure – the ability to fly non-stop over several time zones in a few hours had never been possible before. Under natural conditions, humans would only ever experience changes of seconds or minutes in their daily light–dark cycle but, with the advent of jet travel, we were able to jump multiple time zones in an evolutionary instant.

Why is shift-work a problem?

As reviewed earlier (Chapter 3), the circadian clock in the brain needs to be reset to 24 hours each day, and the solar light–dark cycle performs this role. When a shift-worker works overnight, they expose themselves to light at a time when the circadian clock anticipates darkness. The circadian pacemaker interprets light to mean 'daytime' (which would always be the case under natural light conditions) and therefore starts to shift to readapt to the new 'daytime'. It takes a day to shift about 1 hour under real-world conditions, and therefore we would expect it to take 12 days to adapt from a day shift starting at 8 a.m., to a night shift starting at 8 p.m. This is possible in fixed night or day shifts that persist for several weeks at a time. Unfortunately, most shift-workers' schedules change every few days and do not allow enough time to adapt, or are interrupted by days off (when workers tend not to maintain a 'work' schedule), and so the shift-worker either partially adapts or does not adapt at all during the night shifts. Even if they did adapt, they would need to re-adapt to go back to day shifts and the problem would start all over again. A different approach is to have a rotating shift system that changes so rapidly that circadian adaptation cannot occur (e.g., 1–4 days on each shift) which ensures that workers are never adapted to the night shift and are required to work at the time when sleepiness is highest.

The basic problem is that the shift pattern, and therefore the light–dark cycle, change more rapidly than the circadian system can adapt to, resulting in wake (work) and sleep occurring at an inappropriate circadian phase. Trying to sleep at the wrong circadian phase reduces sleep duration, alters the type and quality of sleep, and affects hormone levels and metabolism. Trying to stay awake at night when the circadian clock is signalling the brain to sleep also causes sleepiness and problems with performance, concentration, and memory. Insomnia or excessive sleepiness associated with the night-work schedule for at least a month are the clinical symptoms of shift-work disorder, a formally recognized sleep disorder. An estimated 3.6 million people work shifts in the UK, with 15 million in the US, and many millions more worldwide. The shift-work revolution has by no means ended but is being repeated on an even larger scale in Asia, South America, and Africa as more nations develop their industrial capacity. Access to electricity widens every day which, while bringing commercial and societal advances, also brings with it the concept and complications of night-work. Rural farming communities that based their day around the immutable pattern of dawn and dusk can now, literally overnight, undo thousands of years of human ecology by extending their day and reducing sleep.

In addition to 'traditional' night shift-workers, about one-fifth of the workforce also have their sleep hours dramatically disrupted.

'Early risers', people who have to start work very early, curtail their sleep by not going to bed early enough due to family, social, and other pressures. Many people also work late and long hours, which pushes back bedtime without necessarily pushing back wake time, squeezing the time available for sleep.

Is jetlag real?

Jetlag is essentially the same problem as shift-work except that the desynchrony between circadian rhythms and the light–dark cycle is caused by long-distance travel. As with shift-work, the circadian system cannot adapt to the rapid change in light–dark exposure and the symptoms – insomnia, fatigue, impaired cognition, gastrointestinal problems – persist until the circadian system has adapted to the new destination, which takes approximately one day per time zone. The number of people affected by jetlag is rising rapidly – hundreds of millions of travellers now fly internationally each year.

How well you adapt to the new time zone depends on your individual circadian pacemaker. About three-quarters of the population have a circadian clock that naturally delays (has a period slightly longer than 24 hours), which means that they have to advance their clock each day to become synchronized. The other quarter have a circadian period less than 24 hours, which means that their clock is slightly advanced and needs to be reset later each day. Travelling westwards requires a delay shift in order to adapt, and travelling eastwards needs an advance shift. In order to work out the adaptation direction, think of what the people are doing now in the time zone you are travelling to: if you are in London having an early evening meal, people in New York are having lunch – their activities are delayed by 5 hours compared to London, and therefore a delay shift is required to adapt to a westward trip from London to New York. At the same time, people in Mumbai are going to bed, as they are set 6 hours earlier compared to London, and therefore an advance shift is needed to

Box 5: Jetlag and sports performance

In 1995, US researchers analysed baseball results based on the direction of travel of the visiting teams. They hypothesized that teams travelling west, whose players would on average be shifting in the same direction as their body clock, would be more successful than teams travelling east, the majority of whom would be going against their natural clock time. Their theory was confirmed. When the visiting team travelled west, 'with' their body clock, they won 44% of the games. When the visiting team travelled east, 'against' their body clock, they won only 37% of their games. Not travelling was best – the visiting team won 46% of games when they did not cross time zones (gamblers take note!). Ideally, sports teams should get to the new venue well ahead of time to reset their body clocks – where milliseconds can mean the difference between winning and losing, full circadian adaptation is a must.

adapt to Indian time. As most people have a circadian clock that naturally delays each day, most people find it easier to adapt to westward travel. On the other hand, those with a naturally advancing clock will find it easier to adapt to eastward travel. These differences can have measurable effects on the rate of adaptation of sleep, alertness, and performance patterns.

Managing shift-work and jetlag

Minimizing the sleep disruption and circadian desynchrony associated with shift-work and jetlag is complex but possible. While it is beyond the scope of this book to review solutions in detail, some general principles apply. Shift duration should be minimized, with night shifts as short as possible. The number of consecutive night shifts should be minimized, and rotating shifts should cycle in a delay direction, that is, from morning, to evening, to night shifts. As much time off as possible should be given after night shifts to maximize recovery sleep. The main problem for night shift-workers is their inability to sleep during the day. Shift-workers should get home and sleep as soon as possible after the shift ends (not watch TV or answer email) and should use an eye-mask and ear-plugs and switch off the telephone when sleeping. Caffeine can be helpful for maintaining alertness on the job, but it should be used 'little and often' and stopped at least 5 hours before the planned sleep time (Chapter 8). Appropriately timed light and dark exposure can be used to facilitate adaptation to the shift, but the shift pattern will determine the exact advice; all schedules should be designed to maximize sleep and alertness, however.

Unlike shift-work, most episodes of jetlag are isolated and the direction and number of time zones are predictable. It is therefore possible to design countermeasures, such as scheduled light–dark exposure, to increase the rate of adaptation and reduce the number of days taken to re-entrain to the new time zone. Such schedules require understanding of the phase response curve (PRC) for light in order to time light and dark exposure appropriately (Figure 14). As a general rule, when normally entrained, light exposure from 18:00–6:00 hours will delay the circadian pacemaker (required to adapt to westward travel), and light from 6:00–18:00 hours will advance the clock (required for eastward travel). The phase-delaying and -advancing effects of the light are greatest about 3 hours before and 3 hours after 6:00 hours, respectively. As the clock shifts to adapt, however, so does the PRC, and so shifts in the windows for advancing and delaying the clock also need to be calculated. Often travellers will be advised to 'get on the new time zone as quickly as possible', but, while this advice is valid for some trips, it can in fact make the jetlag worse in some cases by recommending light exposure at a time that will shift the clock in the opposite direction to that desired. A more sophisticated approach is required using appropriately timed light exposure, natural or indoor, and light avoidance (e.g. dark sunglasses or napping) and, with the right knowledge, adaptation to the new time zone can be accelerated even for very complex travel itineraries.

Consider a flight from New York to London leaving at 7:00 hours (Figure 14a). The flight lasts 7 hours and arrives in London at 19:00 local time, given the 5-hour difference in time zones. In order to adapt to UK time, people travelling eastward from the US need to advance their circadian system. According to the PRC, light exposure at 19:00 New York time will cause a phase delay, opposite to that required. When the traveller arrives in London, however, minimal circadian adaptation has yet taken place, and therefore he remains set to US time (it is 14:00 according to his internal body clock). Consultation of the PRC for 14:00 shows that light at this time and for the next 4 hours will cause a phase advance. In fact, light exposure during the entire duration of the flight is also at the correct time to cause a phase advance. The advice to the traveller is therefore to expose himself to as much light as possible for the entire flight and for the first 4 hours in London, retiring to bed at 23:00 London time and avoiding the phase-delaying effects of light that would begin at this time (Figure 14a).

Now consider the same flight but leaving New York at 19:00, arriving in London at 7:00 (Figure 14b). Again, a 5-hour phase advance is required to adapt to the new time. Most people would follow the same plan as the daytime flight and expose themselves to light upon landing in London. Closer inspection, however, reveals that this plan will send the circadian system in the wrong direction and prevent adaptation to London time. When landing in London at 7:00, the circadian system is still synchronized to US time, that is, 2:00. Light exposure at this time causes a particularly robust phase delay, the opposite direction to that required. It is therefore necessary to avoid light at this time, and for the next 4 hours, until the PRC predicts that light will start to cause a phase advance (6:00 New York time, or 11:00 London time; Figure 14b). The advice to the traveller in this case is to avoid light during the entire flight and for the first 4 hours in

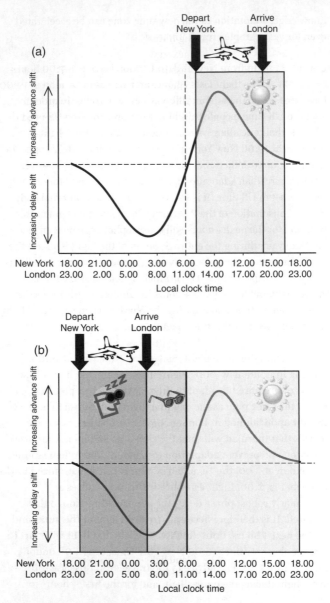

London by sleeping, using an eye-mask, or wearing dark sunglasses, and then exposing himself to as much light as possible from 11:00 in London. The next day, light would be avoided before 9:00 and sought after 9:00, assuming that the clock has delayed by 2 hours, and so on until synchronization is complete. Any schedule can be assessed in this way and by careful use of light exposure, natural or indoor, and light avoidance (dark sunglasses will suffice if not asleep or in the dark), adaptation to the new time zone can be significantly enhanced.

What does shift-work do to health?

The damaging effects of shift-work on health and wellbeing are becoming better understood. Shift-workers experience sleep problems, fatigue, poor performance and memory, gastrointestinal problems, and greater risk of accidents and injuries, and have increased long-term risk of cardiovascular disease, diabetes, and some types of cancer.

Accidents and injuries while working on night shifts present the most immediate health risk to shift-workers. Many high-profile industrial accidents occurred at night, for example Exxon Valdez (midnight), Chernobyl (1:30 a.m.), Three Mile Island (4 a.m.), and the risk of injury in industrial settings is on average about 30% higher for night shift compared to day shifts. This risk is exacerbated with the number of consecutive night shifts and the duration of the shift (Figure 13).

14. How to time light to manage jetlag. Light will shift the clock forward (advance) or backward (delay) depending on the time of day of exposure, and the magnitude and direction of the shift is described by the phase response curve (black line). Light from 18:00–6:00 hours will cause a delay; light from 6:00 to 18:00 hours will cause an advance. The opposite is the case for darkness, or light avoidance. Once these properties of light, and light avoidance, are understood, light–dark plans can be developed to maximize adaptation to a new time zone to avoid jetlag (see text)

Box 6: Shift-work and jetlag in space ships and submarines

Space missions and submarines provide unique challenges to sleep and circadian rhythms, and sleepiness-related accidents in such dangerous environments are of concern.

Astronauts sleep only 5–6 hours per night in space due to excitement, workload, heat, noise, and lack of gravity. Sleeping pills are the most commonly used drugs in space, and individual caffeine stashes are carefully monitored. Astronauts' circadian systems can become disrupted by extraterrestrial light patterns. Orbiting the Earth takes 90 minutes, and imposes a 90-minute light–dark cycle as the Sun goes in and out of view. This is too short for the clock to entrain to, and so a 24-hour light–dark cycle therefore needs to be generated in order to maintain entrainment. Energy restrictions limit the available light to no more than indoor room light. In addition, astronauts sometimes work challenging schedules, requiring 12-hour 'slam' shifts from day to night, or require living on a ~23.5-hour 'day' to ensure meeting launch and return dates. Some of these challenges are also present on Earth: the ground controllers of the recent Mars Phoenix Lander mission had to live on a Martian day – 24.66 hours – during the 3-month mission in order to optimize communication. Countermeasures – particularly appropriately timed light exposure – are being tested on the ground as well as in space, to provide a stronger circadian signal and a direct alerting effect, especially before dangerous activities like 'space walks'.

Similar considerations are needed for submariner crews. Travelling around the planet underwater obviously restricts access to natural light–dark cycles and, even with artificial light, submariners' circadian clocks can sometimes 'free-run' on their own individual internal time. Some work or 'watch' schedules also make it difficult for the circadian clock to become synchronized which will disrupt sleep, increase sleepiness, and reduce performance – exactly the opposite to that required. Developing schedules using sleep and circadian principles is vital for these highly dangerous, life-threatening environments.

The risk does not end when the work shift ends, however; the drive home from work is a particularly vulnerable time for a drowsy-driving crash as workers have been awake for a long time and are driving when the circadian system is promoting sleep. In a study of US junior doctor crashes, there was a 2.3-fold increase in the odds of having a crash on the drive home from a 24-hour shift as compared to when driving home from a non-24-hour shift. The lack of circadian adaptation combined with poor-quality daytime sleep increases night-worker sleepiness dramatically and places both the shift-worker and the public at risk of sleepiness-related accidents.

Shift-work also has long-term health consequences. Epidemiological studies have demonstrated that working night shifts is associated with a higher risk of cardiovascular disease, type II diabetes, and some types of cancer. While these studies cannot address the exact mechanism of disease, the light exposure, sleep restriction, and circadian rhythm disruption associated with shift-work are likely to underlie the health risks.

First, shift-workers often eat at the 'wrong' circadian phase, during the night, when the body is not equipped to metabolize food efficiently. Higher levels of insulin, glucose, and fats are present in the blood after eating a meal at night as compared to eating the same meal in the day. Chronic elevation of insulin, glucose, and fats is symptomatic of insulin resistance and metabolic syndrome, and this is a risk factor for type II diabetes and heart disease; only a few days of simulated shift-work in the laboratory can make a young, healthy subject look like a diabetic. Furthermore, the reduced sleep duration inherent in shift-workers also alters metabolism, including changing the ratio of the hormones leptin and ghrelin which promotes increased appetite and food intake following sleep restriction (Chapter 7).

Finally, recent studies have shown that nearly all of our organs, including the liver, heart, pancreas, kidneys, and lungs, are capable of generating their own circadian rhythms in addition to those generated by the clock in the brain. Proper synchronization between these internal rhythms is probably as important as synchronization with the external world for maintaining metabolic function. It makes intuitive sense that the circadian clocks in the oesophagus, stomach, pancreas, intestine, liver, kidney, and bladder must be synchronized together in order to work properly. These peripheral rhythms appear to be more sensitive to non-light time cues, such as meal timing, than the brain, and given the inconsistent exposure to both light and non-light time cues experienced by shift-workers, their internal circadian rhythm organization will become perturbed. The consequences of such disruption are not yet known, although rodents kept on simulated shift-work and jetlag schedules die younger than animals kept on regular sleep–wake and light–dark cycles.

Shift-work, jetlag, and cancer

The relationship between shift-work and cancer risk has received much attention of late. A number of epidemiological studies (although not all) report around a 50% increased risk of breast cancer in shift-working women who regularly worked overnight and in flight attendants who routinely travelled across time zones. After reviewing the available evidence, the World Health Organization stated in 2007 that 'shift-work that involves circadian disruption is probably carcinogenic to humans', placing shift-work in the same category as ultraviolet light and diesel engine exhausts (Group 2A; probable carcinogen). Shortly thereafter, the Danish government compensated several dozen shift-workers and flight attendants with breast cancer on occupational grounds. There is also evidence for a modest increase in risk of colorectal cancer in female shift-workers, and for increased prostate cancer risk in men (although again, not across all studies).

While these epidemiological studies cannot address the mechanism of disease causation, there are a number of theories relating these schedules to cancer risk. In animal studies, light-induced suppression of the pineal hormone melatonin or removal of the pineal gland has been shown to increase tumour growth rates, probably due to increasing nutrient availability for the tumour. Interestingly, totally blind women have about a 50% reduction in breast cancer risk compared to sighted women, and satellite-derived estimates of the intensity of light pollution at night have been correlated with breast (but not lung) cancer risk in women.

Melatonin is also a potent free-radical scavenger which may also play a role in preventing cancer cell damage and proliferation. Cell cycles are under circadian control, and therefore disruption of cellular rhythmicity in peripheral organs by shift-work may make cells more susceptible to damage; notably, tumours in animals kept on a 'jetlag' schedule grow more quickly than those scheduled to a normal light–dark cycle, even in species that do not produce melatonin. Tumours also express circadian rhythms and, in some cases, specifically timed chemotherapy has been shown to be more potent than continuous infusion, probably due to increased susceptibility of tumour cells to damage at different times of day. Core circadian clock genes have also been shown to be involved in tumour development – for example, the *Period2* gene is a potent tumour suppressor, and 'knocking out' *Per2* speeds up tumour growth and host death, and a polymorphism in the *Period3* gene has been associated with increased breast cancer prevalence in pre-menopausal women.

While these epidemiological and animal data suggest a strong association between light exposure, circadian disruption, melatonin, and cancer, there is as yet no direct evidence in humans proving that alteration of melatonin levels, light exposure, or circadian rhythms alters cancer risk, or that taking synthetic melatonin has any effect on cancer risk or proliferation. Further work is ongoing to explore these relationships.

The continuum of sleep and circadian disruption

Sleep disturbance and circadian rhythm disruption are not 'all-or-nothing' states; the degree of disruption is relative and can be considered as a continuum. It may be that changes relative to your own intrinsic sleep, circadian phase, or melatonin levels, regardless of the absolute level, may be what is important. This concept means that, while research has focused on the most extreme examples of sleep and circadian rhythm disorders, relatively small but chronic day-to-day changes in sleep and circadian phase may also have measurable effects on health that we are yet to understand. Think of the variability in your own sleep–wake cycle; how does your sleep change from work days to non-work days? How often do you stay up especially late or get up especially early for something? How often is your sleep pattern changed unexpectedly by illness, children, pets, noise and light pollution, stress, parties, and so on? Keep in mind that changes in sleep–wake patterns also mean changes in light–dark exposure which shifts the timing of your circadian clock.

The question becomes, therefore, what is the health risk associated with these day-to-day changes? Even though these changes are small, they have occurred only very recently in our evolutionary development and could be considered 'unnatural' – prior to electric light, our ancestors would have had a sleep pattern much more closely related to the natural light–dark cycle. 'Midnight' and 'midday' are not accurate terms in relation to our sleep–wake cycles any more, and we often do not even go to bed until after the 'middle of the night'. For example, melatonin production usually begins at 9–10 p.m. under dim light conditions. Staying awake, even in relatively dim indoor room light, suppresses melatonin output significantly and shortens melatonin production. Consistent with shift-workers (who are an extreme example of 'short' – zero – sleep duration at night), women who report sleeping most (≥9 hours per night) have the lowest breast cancer risk as compared to women who report sleeping 7–8 or ≤6 hours per night.

Until more is understood about the impact of sleep deficiency, circadian disruption, and nighttime light exposure on human health, the weight of current evidence points towards the idea that healthy people should get more sleep, have a regular sleep–wake schedule, and minimize exposure to light at night. As a society, we should promote sleep-friendly and dark-friendly policies and lifestyles, and we should prioritize, value, and savour our nighttime repose as a time to restore our body, our brain, and our health. Without sleep, we would soon die, and without good sleep, we will die sooner – so sleep tight!

Further reading

Chapter 1: Sleep through the ages

J. A. Hobson, *Sleep* (Scientific American Library Series) (W. H. Freeman, 1995).

N. Kleitman, *Sleep and Wakefulness* (University of Chicago Press, 1939, 1963).

Chapter 2: Sleep generation and regulation – a framework

J. Arendt, *Melatonin and the Mammalian Pineal Gland* (Chapman & Hall, 1995).

D. J. Dijk, 'Regulation and functional correlates of slow wave sleep', *Journal of Clinical Sleep Medicine*, 2009, 5 (2 Suppl): S6–15. Available at: http://www.ncbi.nlm.nih.gov/pmc/articles/ PMC2824213/pdf/jcsm.5.2S.S6.pdf

D. J. Dijk and S. W. Lockley, 'Integration of human sleep–wake regulation and circadian rhythmicity', *Journal of Applied Physiology*, 2002, 92 (2): 852–62. Available at: http://jap. physiology.org/content/92/2/852.full.pdf

R. G. Foster and L. Kreitzman, *Rhythms of Life: The Biological Clocks that Control the Daily Lives of Every Living Thing* (Profile Books, 2004).

J. A. Hobson, *Dreaming: A Very Short Introduction* (Oxford University Press, 2005).

S. N. Peirson, S. Halford, and R. G. Foster, 'The evolution of irradiance detection: melanopsin and the non-visual opsins', *Philosophical Transactions of the Royal Society London, B:*

Biological Sciences, 2009, 364 (1531): 2849–65. Available at:
http://www.ncbi.nlm.nih.gov/pmc/articles/PMC2781857/pdf/
rstb20090050.pdf

Chapter 3: The sleeping brain

C. Cirelli, 'The genetic and molecular regulation of sleep: from fruit
  flies to humans', *Nature Reviews Neuroscience*, 2009, 10 (8):
  549–60. Available at: http://www.ncbi.nlm.nih.gov/pmc/articles/
  PMC2767184/pdf/nihms152790.pdf

A. Crocker and A. Sehgal, 'Genetic analysis of sleep', *Genes and
  Development*, 2010, 24 (12): 1220–35. Available at: http://
  www.ncbi.nlm.nih.gov/pmc/articles/PMC2885658/pdf/
  1220.pdf

P. M. Fuller, C. B. Saper, and J. Lu, 'The pontine REM switch: past and
  present', *Journal of Physiology*, 2007, 584 (Pt 3): 735–41. Available
  at: http://www.ncbi.nlm.nih.gov/pmc/articles/PMC2276987/pdf/
  tjp0584-0735.pdf

M. Hastings, J. S. O'Neill, and E. S. Maywood, 'Circadian clocks:
  regulators of endocrine and metabolic rhythms', *Journal of
  Endocrinology*, 2007, 195 (2): 187–98. Available at: http://joe.
  endocrinology-journals.org/content/195/2/187.full.pdf

J. M. Krueger, D. M. Rector, S. Roy, H. P. Van Dongen, G. Belenky, and
  J. Panksepp, 'Sleep as a fundamental property of neuronal
  assemblies', *Nature Reviews Neuroscience*, 2008, 9 (12): 910–19.
  Available at: http://www.ncbi.nlm.nih.gov/pmc/articles/
  PMC2586424/pdf/nihms78194.pdf

R. W. McCarley, 'Neurobiology of REM and NREM sleep', *Sleep
  Medicine*, 2007, 8 (4): 302–30.

M. O'Shea, *The Brain: A Very Short Introduction* (Oxford University
  Press, 2006).

C. B. Saper, P. M. Fuller, N. P. Pedersen, J. Lu, and T. E. Scammell,
  'Sleep state switching', *Neuron*, 2010, 68 (6): 1023–42.

Chapter 4: The reasons for sleep

R. Allada and J. M. Siegel, 'Unearthing the phylogenetic roots of sleep',
  Current Biology, 2008, 18 (15): R670–79. Available at: http://
  www.ncbi.nlm.nih.gov/pmc/articles/PMC2899675/pdf/
  nihms213677.pdf

P. McNamara, R. A. Barton, and C. L. Nunn (eds.), *Evolution of Sleep: Phylogenetic and Functional Perspectives* (Cambridge University Press, 2009).

E. Mignot, 'Why we sleep: the temporal organization of recovery', *PLoS Biology*, 2008, 6 (4): e106. Available at: http://www.ncbi.nlm.nih.gov/pmc/articles/PMC2689703/pdf/pbio.0060106.pdf

V. M. Savage and G. B. West, 'A quantitative, theoretical framework for understanding mammalian sleep', *Proceedings of the National Academy of Sciences USA*, 2007, 104 (3): 1051–6. Available at: http://www.ncbi.nlm.nih.gov/pmc/articles/PMC1783362/pdf/zpq1051.pdf

R. Stickgold and M. P. Walker, 'Sleep-dependent memory consolidation and reconsolidation', *Sleep Medicine*, 2007, 8 (4): 331–43. Available at: http://www.ncbi.nlm.nih.gov/pmc/articles/PMC2680680/pdf/nihms24106.pdf

Chapter 5: The seven ages of sleep

R. Ferber, *Solve Your Child's Sleep Problems*, 2nd edn. (Fireside, 2006).

M. H. Hagenauer, J. I. Perryman, T. M. Lee, and M. A. Carskadon, 'Adolescent changes in the homeostatic and circadian regulation of sleep', *Developmental Neuroscience*, 2009, 31 (4): 276–84. Available at: http://www.ncbi.nlm.nih.gov/pmc/articles/PMC2820578/pdf/dne0031-0276.pdf

I. Iglowstein, O. G. Jenni, L. Molinari, and R. H. Largo, 'Sleep duration from infancy to adolescence: reference values and generational trends', *Pediatrics*, 2003 Feb, 111 (2): 302–7. Available at: http://pediatrics.aappublications.org/content/111/2/302.full.pdf

J. L. Martin and S. Ancoli-Israel, 'Sleep disturbances in long-term care', *Clinical Geriatric Medicine*, 2008, 24 (1): 39–50, vi. Available at: http://www.ncbi.nlm.nih.gov/pmc/articles/PMC2215778/pdf/nihms36700.pdf

M. L. Moline, L. Broch, R. Zak, and V. Gross, 'Sleep in women across the life cycle from adulthood through menopause', *Sleep Medicine Review*, 2003, 7 (2): 155–77.

A. B. Neikrug and S. Ancoli-Israel, 'Sleep disorders in the older adult: a mini-review', *Gerontology*, 2010, 56 (2): 181–9. Available at:

http://www.ncbi.nlm.nih.gov/pmc/articles/PMC2842167/pdf/
ger0056-0181.pdf

R. F. Riemersma-van der Lek, D. F. Swaab, J. Twisk, E. M. Hol,
W. J. Hoogendijk, and E. J. Van Someren, 'Effect of bright light and
melatonin on cognitive and noncognitive function in elderly
residents of group care facilities: a randomized controlled trial',
Journal of the American Medical Association, 2008, 299 (22):
2642–55. Available at: http://jama.ama-assn.org/content/
299/22/2642.full.pdf

Chapter 6: When sleep suffers

American Academy of Sleep Medicine, *International Classification of
Sleep Disorders* (ICSD-2), 2nd edn. (Rochester, MN: American
Academy of Sleep Medicine, 2005).

L. Epstein and S. Mardon, *The Harvard Medical School Guide to a
Good Night's Sleep* (McGraw-Hill, 2006).

S. Wilson and D. Nutt, *Sleep Disorders* (Oxford Psychiatry Library)
(Oxford University Press, 2008).

Chapter 7: Sleep and health

F. P. Cappuccio, M. A. Miller, and S. W. Lockley (eds.), *Sleep, Health
and Society: From Aetiology to Public Health* (Oxford University
Press, 2010).

K. L. Knutson, K. Spiegel, P. Penev, and E. Van Cauter, 'The metabolic
consequences of sleep deprivation', *Sleep Medicine Review*, 2007,
11 (3): 163–78. Available at: http://www.ncbi.nlm.nih.gov/pmc/
articles/PMC1991337/pdf/nihms25263.pdf

K. Wulff, S. Gatti, J. G. Wettstein, and R. G. Foster, 'Sleep and
circadian rhythm disruption in psychiatric and neurodegenerative
disease', *Nature Reviews Neuroscience*, 2010, 11 (8): 589–99.

Chapter 8: Sleep and society

F. P. Cappuccio, A. Bakewell, F. M. Taggart, G. Ward, C. Ji, J. P.
Sullivan, M. Edmunds, R. Pounder, C. P. Landrigan, S. W. Lockley,
and E. Peile, for the Warwick EWTD Working Group. 'Implementing
a 48-hour EWTD-compliant rota for junior doctors in the UK does

not compromise patients' safety: assessor-blind pilot comparison', *Quarterly Journal of Medicine*, 2009, 102 (4): 271–82. Available at: http://www.ncbi.nlm.nih.gov/pmc/articles/PMC2659599/pdf/hcp004.pdf

C. A. Czeisler, 'Medical and genetic differences in the adverse impact of sleep loss on performance: ethical considerations for the medical profession', *Transactions of the American Clinical and Climatological Association*, 2009, 120: 249–85. Available at: http://www.ncbi.nlm.nih.gov/pmc/articles/PMC2744509/pdf/tacca120000249.pdf

F. Danner and B. Phillips, 'Adolescent sleep, school start times, and teen motor vehicle crashes', *Journal of Clinical Sleep Medicine*, 2008, 4 (6): 533–5. Available at: http://www.ncbi.nlm.nih.gov/pmc/articles/PMC2603528/pdf/jcsm.4.6.533.pdf

C. B. Jones, J. Dorrian, and S. M. Rajaratnam, 'Fatigue and the criminal law', *Industrial Health*, 2005, 43 (1): 63–70. Available at: http://www.jstage.jst.go.jp/article/indhealth/43/1/63/_pdf

A. C. Levine, J. Adusumilli, and C. P. Landrigan, 'Effects of reducing or eliminating resident work shifts over 16 hours: a systematic review', *Sleep*, 2010, 33 (8): 1043–53. Available at: http://www.ncbi.nlm.nih.gov/pmc/articles/PMC2910534/pdf/aasm.33.8.1043. pdf

R. P. Millman, 'Excessive sleepiness in adolescents and young adults: causes, consequences, and treatment strategies', *Pediatrics*, 2005, 115 (6): 1774–86. Available at: http://pediatrics.aappublications.org/content/115/6/1774.full.pdf

J. L. Temple, 'Caffeine use in children: what we know, what we have left to learn, and why we should worry', *Neuroscience and Biobehavioral Reviews*, 2009, 33 (6): 793–806. Available at: http://www.ncbi.nlm.nih.gov/pmc/articles/PMC2699625/pdf/nihms117089.pdf

S. J. Williams, *Sleep and Society: Sociological Ventures into the Un(known)* (Routledge, 2005).

Chapter 9: The 24-hour society

T. Akerstedt and K. P. Wright, 'Sleep loss and fatigue in shift work and shift work disorder', *Sleep Medicine Clinics*, 2009, 4 (2): 257–71. Available at: http://www.ncbi.nlm.nih.gov/pmc/articles/PMC2904525/pdf/nihms215779.pdf

J. Arendt, 'Jetlag and shift work: (2) Therapeutic use of melatonin', *Journal of the Royal Society of Medicine*, 1999, 92 (8): 402–5. Available at: http://www.ncbi.nlm.nih.gov/pmc/articles/PMC1297315/pdf/jrsocmed00006-0022.pdf

P. Cinzano, F. Falchi, and C. D. Elvidge, 'The first world atlas of the artificial night sky brightness', *Monthly Notices of the Royal Astronomical Society*, 2001, 328: 689–707. Available at: http://www.lightpollution.it/cinzano/download/0108052.pdf

C. I. Eastman and H. J. Burgess, 'How to travel the world without jet lag', *Sleep Medicine Clinics*, 2009, 4(2): 241–55. Available at: http://www.ncbi.nlm.nih.gov/pmc/articles/PMC2829880/pdf/nihms166069.pdf

S. Folkard and P. Tucker, 'Shift work, safety and productivity', Occupational Medicine (London), 2003, 53 (2): 95–101. Available at: http://occmed.oxfordjournals.org/content/53/2/95.full.pdf

A. Knutsson, 'Health disorders of shift workers', Occupational Medicine (London), 2003, 53 (2): 103–8. Available at: http://occmed.oxfordjournals.org/content/53/2/103.full.pdf

R. L. Sack, D. Auckley, R. R. Auger, M. A. Carskadon, K. P. Wright, Jr, M. V. Vitiello, and I. V. Zhdanova, 'Circadian rhythm sleep disorders: Part I, basic principles, shift work and jetlag disorders', *Sleep*, 2007, 30 (11): 1460–83. Available at: http://www.ncbi.nlm.nih.gov/pmc/articles/PMC2082105/pdf/aasm.30.11.1460.pdf

R. G. Stevens, D. E. Blask, G. C. Brainard, J. Hansen, S. W. Lockley, I. Provencio, M. S. Rea, and L. Reinlib, 'Meeting report: the role of environmental lighting and circadian disruption in cancer and other diseases', *Environmental Health Perspectives*, 2007, 115 (9): 1357–62. Available at: http://www.ncbi.nlm.nih.gov/pmc/articles/PMC1964886/pdf/ehp0115-001357.pdf

Websites

www.understandingsleep.org
Website of the Sleep and Health Education Program, Division of Sleep Medicine, Harvard Medical School, Boston, MA, USA

www.ncbi.nlm.nih.gov/pubmed/
Website of the US National Library of Medicine National Institutes of Health database of scientific papers

Index

Index

Sleep

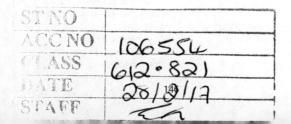

162

Expand your collection of
VERY SHORT INTRODUCTIONS

MEMORY
A Very Short Introduction
Michael J. Benton

Why do we remember events from our childhood as if they
happened yesterday, but not what we did last week? Why does
our memory seem to work well sometimes and not others?
What happens when it goes wrong? Can memory be improved
or manipulated, by psychological techniques or even 'brain
implants'? How does memory grow and change as we age?
And what of so-called 'recovered' memories? This book brings
together the latest research in neuroscience and psychology,
and weaves in case-studies, anecdotes, and even literature
and philosophy, to address these and many other important
questions about the science of memory - how it works,
and why we can't live without it.

www.oup.com/vsi